THE FIVE TIBETANS

"Inspired and clear, *The Five Tibetans* makes a worthy contribution to body-mind wellness and longevity."

MEHMET OZ, M.D.,
PROFESSOR OF SURGERY AT COLUMBIA UNIVERSITY,
DIRECTOR OF THE CARDIOVASCULAR INSTITUTE &
COMPLEMENTARY MEDICINE PROGRAM AT NEW YORK–
PRESBYTERIAN HOSPITAL, AND HOST OF *THE DR. OZ SHOW*

"Chris Kilham's *The Five Tibetans* is a time-honored classic that belongs in every yoga library. A true yogi, Chris's voice is strong, sensitive, and clear; his calling deep and genuine."

DEEPAK CHOPRA, M.D.,
WORLD-RENOWNED AUTHORITY ON MIND-BODY HEALING,
BESTSELLING AUTHOR, AND FOUNDER OF THE CHOPRA CENTER
FOR WELLBEING

"I know hundreds of individuals who swear by this practice on a daily basis. Chris's ability to translate this powerful teaching in a simple way has led to great self-transformation."

JONNY KEST,
CREATOR OF SLOWBURN YOGA
AND DIRECTOR OF THE
JONNY KEST YOGA TEACHER TRAINING PROGRAM

"In *The Five Tibetans,* Chris Kilham offers a simple yet profound practice that promotes health and longevity, is centering, and leads to peace of mind. Chris is a jewel among men!"

NICKI DOANE,
AUTHORIZED ASHTANGA YOGA TEACHER AND
CODIRECTOR OF MAYA YOGA STUDIOS

"The Five Tibetans are a perfect practice for a balanced life and a healthy body."

EDDIE MODESTINI,
CERTIFIED IYENGAR AND ASHTANGA YOGA
TEACHER AND CODIRECTOR OF MAYA YOGA STUDIOS

"This book is packed full of expert information . . . clear, concise, and easy to understand . . . a wealth of information and advice from many years of teaching and personal experiences . . . a wonderful way to start or end your day."

TCM REVIEWS

"Kilham brings to the Five Tibetans beautifully written chapters about kundalini, the chakras, and an especially insightful instruction on the role of breathing while doing each rite. Excellent and recommended."

HINDUISM TODAY

THE FIVE TIBETANS

Five Dynamic Exercises for Health, Energy, and Personal Power

CHRISTOPHER S. KILHAM

Healing Arts Press
Rochester, Vermont • Toronto, Canada

Healing Arts Press
One Park Street
Rochester, Vermont 05767
www.HealingArtsPress.com

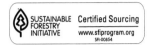

Text stock is SFI certified

Healing Arts Press is a division of Inner Traditions International

Note to the reader: This book is intended as an informational guide. The remedies, approaches, and techniques described herein are meant to supplement, and not to be a substitute for, professional medical care or treatment. They should not be used to treat a serious ailment without prior consultation with a qualified health care professional.

Library of Congress Cataloging-in-Publication Data
Kilham, Christopher.
  The five tibetans : five dynamic exercises for health, energy, and personal power / Christopher S. Kilham.
    p. cm.
  Summary: "New edition of the popular yoga classic"—Provided by publisher.
  ISBN 978-1-59477-444-7 (pbk.) — ISBN 978-1-59477-808-7 (ebook)
  1. Hatha yoga. I. Title.
  RA781.7.K52 2011
  613.7'046—dc23

                                                                    2011020220

Printed and bound in the United States by Lake Book Manufacturing
The text stock is SFI certified. The Sustainable Forestry Initiative® program promotes sustainable forest management.

10 9 8 7 6 5 4 3

Text design and layout by Virginia Scott Bowman
This book was typeset in Garamond Premier Pro with Warnock Pro and Futura as display typefaces

Photograph on page viii by David Johnston, Johnston Photography
Illustration on page 18 by Christina Camphausen
Photographs of the Five Tibetans by Janice Fullman

To send correspondence to the author of this book, mail a first-class letter to the author c/o Inner Traditions • Bear & Company, One Park Street, Rochester, VT 05767, and we will forward the communication.

This new edition of The Five Tibetans
is dedicated to the thousands of people
who have practiced these postures in my yoga classes,
to my wife Zoe Helene, and
to the yogis, mystics, shamans, and teachers
around the world who have inspired me.

CONTENTS

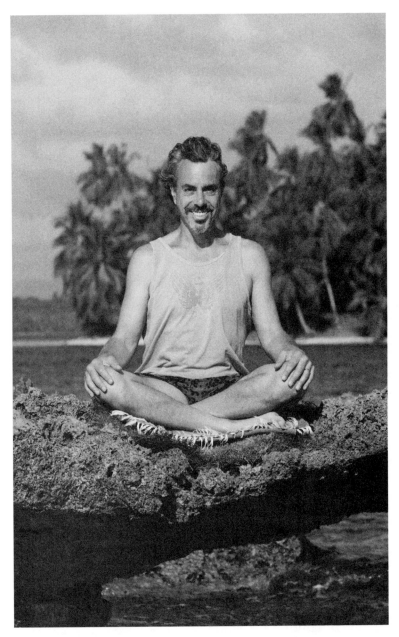

The author on a coral outcropping above the blue waters
of the San Blas Islands, Panama, 2011.

INTRODUCTION TO THE NEW EDITION

One of my favorite quotes from a spiritual scripture says, "This will all seem like a brief flash of heat lightning on a summer day." That is one of the great mysteries of life, that time flashes by at a tremendous rate. Days turn into months, months turn into years, and years quickly multiply into decades. Sometimes we begin something, and at a certain point we stop to consider that we've been involved with that activity for a long time.

So it goes with the Five Tibetans. I encountered them in 1976, began to practice them daily in 1978, and now, thirty-five years later, I am still practicing these methods every day. Except for the rare occasion when I am flying someplace around the clock, I practice yoga each morning and always finish with the Five Tibetans. When I first took them up, it was hard to say for sure what benefits I would derive or how long I would enjoy making them part of my life. Decades later, I can say with certainty that the benefits derived from practicing the Five Tibetans are many, and I have every intention of making them an integral part of my daily life until I can no longer do so.

As a medicine hunter, I travel the world in search of traditional remedies that can help alleviate human suffering, remedies that can be used in place of dangerous, potentially lethal pharmaceuticals. As part of this work, I find myself in many countries, often in very remote places. In all my travels, the Five Tibetans have been my companions. I have practiced these methods in Vanuatu South Pacific; in Siberia; Morocco; the Peruvian, Brazilian, and Ecuadorian Amazon; high up in the Indian Himalayas; in the Syrian desert; along Xinjiang's Naladi grasslands; on the Mexican coast; and in countless cities from Kathmandu to Shanghai to Marrakech to Moscow to London to Accra. I have practiced them in hotels, on beaches, on stone patios, in native shacks, on boat docks, in forests, on mountains, and in airports. As the Johnny Cash song says, "I've been everywhere." And so have the Five Tibetans.

The Five Tibetans book has been busy too, starting from its publication in the United States, to its current publication in twenty languages and more than twenty-two countries. I have found *The Five Tibetans* in bookshops in London, Amsterdam, Mumbai, Mexico, and many other places. I never could have imagined such a positive reception. *The Five Tibetans* is the little book that just keeps on going. It sits on coffee tables, bookshelves, counters, and bedside tables all over the globe. How wonderful is that?

One of the claims made about the Five Tibetans is that they are youth enhancers. When I first wrote this book, I frankly admitted that I did not actually know one way or another if this was true, but I hoped to find out. Now, decades later, I can say that the Five Tibetans definitely help to maintain more youthful strength, flexibility, balance, circulation, energy, endurance, and stamina. I also credit them with helping to keep me mentally sharp. That's not bad at all for a ten-minute daily practice. Despite this, I'm still aging, looking older than I did decades ago, and going through various processes of change as the years melt by. Any of us who live long enough will age. That is a guarantee. But, yes, I can state that, as advertised, the Five Tibetans make a difference in at least slowing down the aging process. And this is a mighty thing.

Throughout the ages, for as far back as history can recount, people have sought health secrets of various types, from exotic elixirs to mystic ceremonies to tantric rituals, foul-smelling concoctions, viper venoms, odd foods, breathing exercises, dances, and countless other means. The very practice of yoga, in all its forms, is designed to engender greater physical, mental, and spiritual health while advancing consciousness and opening the practitioner to broader awareness of innate divinity. Among the offerings available in the vast buffet of yogic practices, the Five Tibetans hold a special place. They are dynamic, they are accessible to most people, they produce results that you can feel, and they add vitality to your life. If you can allocate only ten minutes a day for yoga, practice the Five Tibetans.

When I think back over the years, I smile at all the places and times I have practiced these methods. And I am grateful that during most of the thirty-seven years I taught yoga, I turned thousands of people on to the Five Tibetans. While I have no idea how many of them still practice these methods today, I feel that I have been a good and worthy emissary. My belief about yoga is that we do not find it; yoga finds us. As a persistent and perennial current of spiritual dynamism, yoga uses us to spread itself, to broaden its reach, to touch the lives of others, to keep itself going. Many years ago, the Five Tibetans came to me. They caught my imagination. I started to practice them. Eventually I became their ardent advocate. I spread the word far and wide. Today, I am still working on their behalf, still spreading the word, still sharing the methods.

Except for this new introduction, nothing has changed in this book, including the photos that show me as a much younger man. But I still practice yoga for almost two hours daily, I hike almost every day, bodysurf any wave I can find, snowshoe in winter storms, bicycle during the warm season, troop my way through forests and mountains around the globe, and maintain a vigorous life. At least some of this is due to the Five Tibetans. I can say without question that I am indebted to them, am grateful for them, and am deeply honored to share them with the rest of the world. I hope that you will find value in this book, will be inspired by what is written here, and will reap rich benefits from your own personal practice of the Five Tibetans.

CHRIS KILHAM
MASSACHUSETTS, 2011

PREFACE AND ACKNOWLEDGMENTS

I have been profoundly influenced by the Five Tibetans since discovering them in 1976. Now, with the opportunity to write this book, I am able to share what I know about the Five Tibetans and to present other related yogic methods and concepts.

My discovery of yoga seems nothing less than an act of grace. I do not think that I am clever enough to have planned the wonderful adventure that has been mine thanks to yoga and meditation. And I know for sure that I could not have conjured a series of yoga methods as simple and yet as powerful as the Five Tibetans.

The best way I know to express my gratitude and appreciation for yoga and all that it has done for me is to share it—thus this book. I hope you will find it enjoyable and stimulating. I hope it will pique your curiosity and make you want to try the methods described. I wish you great success, whoever you are. Blessings.

⊕

I wish to express my thanks and appreciation to everyone who has attended my yoga classes since I first started to teach, with especially fond remembrance of Janet Perry, my student and friend for fifteen years, who recently died and went on to wherever it is that people go. Every teacher, at least once, should have a student as wonderful as Janet.

Thanks to my mom, who used to get dizzy watching me do the first Tibetan; she was my most ardent supporter since day one. Thanks to Roshi Al and Kristin who always prod me on in my peripatetic yogic wanderings. Thanks also to Steve and Craig, intrepid Yucatan–pyramid climbing companions. Cheers to the Tribal Council Elders. You know who you are.

Thanks to zany photographer Janice Fullman, whose ability to capture me through her lens makes me willing to contort myself for hours in the sand. And thanks to the entire crew at Inner Traditions, especially Ehud Sperling and Estella Arias and Leslie Colket Blair, for supporting my ideas and way of yoga, and for giving me a forum to spread this cosmic propaganda far and wide.

Much love to you all.

1 ABOUT THE FIVE TIBETANS

FIRST EXPERIENCES WITH THE FIVE TIBETANS

In 1976 I was invited to live and teach health classes at the Institute of Mentalphysics, a spiritual retreat center in Joshua Tree, California. Occupying a square mile of land in the high desert, the institute boasts views of both the San Gorgonio and San Jacinto mountains, and is only a mile away from the entrance to Joshua Tree National Monument, a destination for rock climbers and adventure travelers worldwide. Joshua Tree is a place of stunning beauty, abundant nature, spectacular rock formations, and spiritual power. It is a place where people go to revive and rejuvenate themselves, undertake vision quests, and contemplate the grandeur of the natural world. It is a perfect neighbor for the Institute of Mentalphysics.

The Institute of Mentalphysics was founded in the 1930s in Los Angeles by a geographer named Edwin Dingle, a man who, through an extraordinary act of fate, wound up living and studying with a high lama in Tibet for nine months in the 1920s. During his brief time under the tutelage of the Tibetan lama, Dingle learned a series of Tibetan yoga breaths and exercises that would later become the heart of the Mentalphysics curriculum of spiritual practice. The methods he learned and subsequently taught in Los Angeles became very popular. Eventually Dingle commissioned Frank Lloyd Wright to design and help build the Mentalphysics spiritual retreat center. For decades to come the institute served as a mecca for spiritual adherents from all over the world.

At the time that I moved to the institute, there were far fewer students than in its heyday, and only a few residents occupied the center's apartments. One of those, a woman named Rochelle, was a wonderfully vibrant character in her early seventies with a history of experiences that comprised an impressive romp through a who's who of gurus, psychics, sages, adepts, seers, avatars, saints, and wanna-be holy men and women. A perfect blend of curiosity, intelligence, positive attitude, and skepticism, and with an appetite for diverse experiences, Rochelle had tried every major and minor spiritual trip popular at that time, and knew all the secret mantras and supposed inner knowledge of most of them.

Seeing that I was a devoted yoga practitioner, Rochelle gave me a copy of an interesting little book entitled *The Five Rites of Rejuvenation* authored by a man named Peter Kelder and first published in 1939. The book recounted an engaging story about the discovery of five yoga exercises taught to Kelder by a retired British army officer who had learned the exercises from some Tibetan lamas in a monastery in the Himalayas. According to the book, the Five Rites of Rejuvenation were reputed to strengthen the body, enhance energy, regenerate body and mind, and stem the aging process.

Having practiced yoga for six years, I was already familiar with a broad repertoire of methods. Intrigued by Kelder's account of their virtues, I began to include the Five Rites of Rejuvenation in my daily yoga routine. I liked the way they had been discovered, the romance of how they had been introduced to a small number of westerners by the man who had learned them in the Himalayas, and the illustrations of the methods themselves. They were similar in appearance to yoga exercises with which I was already familiar, but they were also different enough that they in no way duplicated other practices in my daily routine.

Of particular interest to me was that the Five Rites of Rejuvenation were more similar to the Tibetan yoga methods taught at Mentalphysics than to any other methods I had previously encountered. It seemed highly likely that, based on the description of the monastic and natural environment from which the Five Rites of Rejuvenation originated, they too were Tibetan *in origin*. I never liked the name "Five Rites of Rejuvenation." I always thought it sounded a little cornball, from a comic book, a little too reminiscent of Charles Atlas and the era of the early 1900s. So I began to refer to the exercises as the Five Tibetans.

After practicing the Five Tibetans for two years, I was convinced that, at the very least, they were extraordinary. Despite the fact that they represented only minutes in a daily yoga regimen that was several hours long, I felt invigorated from practicing them. Whether they are in fact the fountain of youth as rhapsodized in Peter Kelder's book remains to be seen. I'll write a followup when I'm eighty and let you know. At the very least, they do in fact greatly increase strength, energy, and mental alertness. They open up the body/mind energy system and seem to balance energy in a way that I have not experienced with any other individual yoga method or set of yoga practices.

In 1978 I started to teach the Five Tibetans to students in all my yoga classes. Since that time I have personally shared the Five Tibetans with at least several hundred people, if not a thousand or more. In 1985 I included the exercises, listed as the Rejuvenation Series, in my book on yoga therapy and nutrition, entitled *Take Charge of Your Health*. The Five Tibetans were also included in my later book *Inner Power: Secrets from Tibet and the Orient* (1988).

In this present volume you'll find a comprehensive approach to a personal yoga practice using the Five Tibetans as a foundation. Specific information about the human energy system, the chakras, and kundalini meditation will give you a complete context for your practice. Whether or not the Five Tibetans are in fact Tibetan in origin is something we may never ascertain. Perhaps they come from Nepal or northern India. I honestly do not know for sure, nor do I really care. As the story has it, they were shared by Tibetan lamas; beyond that I know nothing of their history. What I do know is that the name "Five Tibetans" has caught on as a more acceptable monicker than the "Five Rites of Rejuvenation." I have seen recently published books in German, French, and other languages that also refer to these same exercises as the Five Tibetans. The name rolls off the tongue more easily than the "Five Kathmandus" or the "Five Uttar Pradeshes."

Personally, I think these exercises are most likely Tibetan in origin. The issue at hand, though, is not the lineage of the Five Tibetans. The point is that we have in these exercises a simple yoga routine that is of immense potential value for those who will clear ten minutes from their day to practice.

A MODIFICATION

I must point out that as soon as I began to practice them I modified the Five Tibetans in one very important way. As described in Peter Kelder's book, the exercises included no specified breathing. I believe this to be either an error or a calculated omission. In my extensive study of yoga methods, I have never encountered any techniques involving movement that did not also involve regulated breathing. All the Indian, Tibetan, and Chinese yoga practices I have ever learned accompany movement with breath. Breathing is an essential aspect of yoga practice. It occurred to me that the lack of information on breathing in Kelder's book may have resulted from a belief, commonly held by occultists and spiritualists in the early 1900s, that only partial truths should be imparted to the uninitiated. This attitude can be recognized in most of the Theosophical writings of that period, as well as in the works of Alice Bailey and other spiritual and occult writers of that era. To an extent, this attitude still prevails.

The justification behind imparting half-truths has to do with the notion that people who are not given personal instruction in powerful yoga methods by a guru or master may cause themselves harm. Or worse, they may crash the hallowed gates of the inner circles of initiated practitioners and may walk off—if they choose to do so—having learned authentic techniques without having given the fealty that so many devotees are obliged to bestow upon gurus and other self-proclaimed masters. Therefore, reasoning goes, give the general public enough information about yoga methods to impart an effect, but reserve some key essentials only for those willing to give life and soul to the guru. I personally find this notion misguided at best and reprobate nonsense at worst.

I believe that if a method is valid and beneficial, it is the duty and obligation of any true teacher to pass full knowledge of that method on to those who are interested. Such knowledge should not be withheld or meted out like a weekly allowance to only those devotees who "prove themselves." Furthermore, there is very little danger in imparting even the most potent yoga methods to anybody at all, because all methods must be practiced with consistency over time to have any profound or lasting effect. Even those people who are truly sincere find it difficult to sustain an ongoing yoga practice. Those who are insincere or who apprehend yoga methods in order to garner power to abuse almost always wind up disappointed, and simply stop practicing. The greatest likelihood is that only those who are practicing for healthy reasons will continue. So there is a process of natural selection fundamental to the nature of yoga practice. Therefore, give people everything. Share all methods and withhold nothing. Those who practice steadily and carefully over time will reap great benefits. Those who don't practice will move on and find other things to occupy their time and interest.

To make up for what was either error or deletion, I carefully added regulated breathing to the Five Tibetans in order to maximize their full power. I am pleased to see that other authors who have promoted these exercises in their own books have followed my lead, including breathing exactly as I have prescribed. Based on more than twenty years of yoga practice and teaching, I have every reason to believe that these exercises are far more beneficial with regulated breathing than without it.

DRAWING FROM THE YOGIC TRADITION

The vast systems of yoga, originating from India and the northern regions of Nepal and Tibet, are thousands of years old. Over the course of time yoga has spread throughout the world. Now you can find yoga classes virtually everywhere. Yoga practice typically involves physical exercise, regulated breathing, and meditation. Of these three categories of activity there are literally thousands of methods for the attainment of radiant health, brilliant mental clarity, and spiritual fulfillment. There are similarities among all yoga systems and there are profound differences. The yoga I practice, for example, is a synthesis of methods from the Kundalini, Tibetan, and Chinese yoga traditions. My practice is strenuous and aerobic, and involves a lot of powerful breathing. This suits my somewhat fiery temperament. Traditional hatha yoga, by contrast, appeals to practitioners who are more interested in a gentler practice that enhances overall health and provides stress relief. All yoga systems have their virtues.

Like any other practice, yoga is not static. It evolves and changes over time according to who is practicing and teaching it. Everyone who goes beyond a cursory exploration of yoga will put their own spin on it. Two teachers may offer the very same methods, but from one what is offered will seem somehow more vital, dynamic, and rich. Because yoga practice is totally experiential, it can never be separated from the person who is practicing or teaching it.

Over the millennia that yoga has developed, adepts have discovered some methods that are more powerful or beneficial to health than others. There are many excellent yoga scriptures and writings that describe these methods. In my own pursuits I have drawn heavily from four traditional yoga texts: the *Siva Samhita*, the *Goraksa Sataka*, the *Hatha Yoga Pradipika*, and *Tibetan Yoga and Secret Doctrines* as translated by Lama Kazi Dawa Samdup. Though the language of these texts is sometimes cumbersome and though the scriptures are filled with religious or cultural references, descriptions of ceremonies, and iconography that are not essential to the methods described, they are outstanding sources of information for the earnest yoga practitioner. Many of the ideas expressed here were gleaned from the pages of those august works. I have personally practiced and taught, for at least several years, every one of the methods or recommendations included in this book. I could not otherwise vouch for their efficacy.

Yoga is not only strengthening and enlightening, it is also highly enjoyable. Yoga practice vivifies the senses and enhances your appreciation of all life. It fills you up if you let it. It can be fun and exhilarating. It makes food taste better. It makes sex feel better. It makes breathing a rich pleasure. Yoga also boosts your sense of humor. You can't diligently practice yoga, honing the clarity of your mind, and fail to be struck by the very humorous—albeit pathetic—predicament we're all in. We find ourselves chained to the wheel of karma (what Jack Kerouac calls "the meat wheel"), going round and round in our own private illusory worlds, struggling to glimpse reality and attain eternal peace. It's funny and maddeningly difficult, and sad too, sometimes. It's also the only game in town, and no one gets out alive.

Yoga helps you rise to the challenge of living. It keeps you from being ground down by circumstance. It puts fire into the body and mind, and leads to being balanced and wise. It makes a lot of sense to practice. In this volume you are given tools to strengthen your body, enhance your health, increase your energy, hone your concentration, and experience the profound power and peace of deep meditation. You don't have to endure ascetic austerities or the rugged Himalayan terrain to get at these teachings. They are accessible without restriction, the way all valid teachings should be.

2 ENERGY, BODY, AND MIND

Humans are incarnate beings, which is to say that we are beings who live in bodies. We are not just our bodies, but we are inseparable from them as far as human life is concerned. There may be other, disembodied life after we have discarded our mortal frames. But a human being is incarnate, and that is the simplest and most basic fact of life.

For some crazy reason, the simplicity of incarnation escapes a lot of people. Or perhaps it's the case that the sheer inability to escape the confines of a body simply makes some people go into serious denial. Some "spiritual" people insist that the body is of little significance. They de-emphasize the body, sometimes regarding it as a vulgar barrier to lofty pursuits, and fix their attention on development of the spirit from the standpoint of the mind. Yet they follow this course while inhabiting a body. I wonder what their experience would be without one? For all we know, there may be trillions of discarnate souls urgently waiting for bodies, lined up with the cosmic equivalent of bakery numbers, just waiting to get in.

On the other side of the same warped coin are the reductionists, people who declare that we are *only* our bodies, nothing more than a clever aggregation of blood, skin, bones, and hair. Among the reductionists there is utter disregard for consciousness because it can't be analyzed under a microscope. Yet lots of important things—like ideas, emotions, love, and wisdom—can't be analyzed under a microscope. Does that mean these things don't exist? Of course not. Who are we to assume that only via diagnostic tools devised by humans can we know what is real and what is not? It's a crazy way to think.

In between the abject silliness of these two extremes is the apparent fact that we are both body and mind, inextricably intertwined. It is in the spirit of this very simple understanding that we can consider the human energy system. The human energy system is the energetic substrate of the human body/mind. It is a system within a system and is nonphysical, though every bit as real as our organs, limbs, and face. The human energy system is similar in design and function to the nervous system in that it runs throughout the entire body and has major and minor pathways. The major confluences of nerves in the body are called plexuses; the equivalent in the human energy system are the chakras, centers of concentrated power. While the nervous system conducts trillions of impulses to keep the body running correctly, the human energy system is the link between the universal source of all intelligence and the human body. Unlike the nervous system, the human energy system extends beyond the boundaries of the physical body. The aura, the energetic sheath that envelops the body and is visible to some people, is part of this system.

The human energy system is an energetic webbing that permeates the entire body. It is the system that empowers the body and energizes and enlivens the mind, providing the energetic foundation upon which the body is built. It is the network through which all life energy flows.

I readily admit that to many people the foregoing statements might seem to be pure fantasy. If the human energy system exists, why doesn't everybody experience it? The truth is that we benefit at all times from the workings of the human energy system, but its activities are so thoroughly integrated into every aspect of our regular, daily living that the human energy system goes largely unnoticed. This is typical of many important aspects of our beings. For example, most people do not consciously experience their spleens or their hypothalamic nuclei. Nonetheless, these parts of the body are diligently at work round the clock, bolstering immunity and integrating peripheral autonomic mechanisms respectively. We typically only notice the symptoms that manifest when some part of the body goes awry.

Although the human energy system is constantly at work, keeping us well connected to the source of all life and intelligence, in order to consciously experience it we have to up the voltage, so to speak. This is where yoga, tai chi, or other forms of meditation come in. Through practice of these mind/body disciplines, the human energy system begins to carry an increasingly strong flow of life energy. As this happens, it becomes easy to feel a steady energetic current coursing through us. Over time it is possible to develop both the flow of energy and one's own sensory acuity to the point that the human energy system can be experienced to a very high degree. It becomes palpable, audible, and visible.

Let me share with you one of my earliest experiences with my own energy system. Back in the summer of 1971 I was an eager neophyte yogi, taking in as many good books on yoga and meditation as I could, practicing yoga postures, and meditating at least twice daily. Before going to bed every evening I would practice nad yoga, a method that is described in detail in the meditation section (chapter 9) of this book. Nad yoga involves listening to the sound current, an audible current of energy that runs through the entire body and that can usually be heard by listening in the area of the head near the right ear. My routine was basically the same every evening. I would get into bed, lie on my back with my body perfectly straight, and listen carefully to the sound. After half an hour or so of practice I would turn over and go to sleep. On one particular evening I got into bed as always and began to listen to the sound current. At first nothing seemed unusual or different. But then the sound started to grow steadily in volume, like a symphony that sounds like one faint instrument far away but gets louder with greater differentiation of sounds as you get closer. Instead of hearing a faint hum or buzz, I heard dozens and dozens of sounds, each one getting progressively louder and more distinct. As the volume and clarity of the sound current steadily increased, I began to feel a gentle hum throughout my entire body, as though all my molecules had been roused from a sound sleep and were starting to dance. As the sound increased, the feeling of vibration in my body increased.

After several minutes of this steady progression of sound and feeling, everything intensified dramatically. Suddenly the sound current was roaring from my feet up through my head as loudly as if a train were running through my bedroom. The sensations in my body went from a gentle hum to a feeling of intense vibration; every cell was wild with energy. Up through the center of my spine a powerful current began to flow. It was as though I was a hollow tube and a concentrated torrent of energy was blasting up through me. The roaring sounds and intense sensations were accompanied by a stunning display of vivid colors shooting through my body. Brilliant explosions of gold, yellow, red, blue, purple, and silver flew upward through my body, completely visible to my interior sight. It was as though the most uproarious Chinese New Year celebration ever was happening inside me, replete with a spectacular fireworks display.

After a few meteoric minutes, the sound, feeling, light, and colors began to subside. I felt elated, ecstatic, extraordinarily alive. This was my introduction to the human energy system, my first substantive encounter with the kundalini energy that operates within us, and my first experience of being able to access that energy through yoga practice. It is worth noting that the event was not at all drug related, and that I had not used any mind-altering substances of any kind for a long period of time prior to that evening. Everything that happened was a result of faithfully practicing a yoga technique.

The point of recounting this story is not to impress you, but to impress *upon* you that when I say you can become familiar with your own energy system in ways that are palpable, audible, and visible, I am not referring to dilute, subtle experiences. The human energy system is a frontier of incalculable dimension. It is a landscape filled with raw power, sound, and light. It is the playground of mystics and yogis. It is an exciting and interesting and occasionally terrifying place to journey. With yoga practice you can not only have extraordinary experiences that are otherwise only available through the use of potent psychedelic drugs, but you can learn to develop a measure of conscious control over the energy that flows through you. It is a worthwhile pursuit.

Consider how many things seem unattainable until you work at them. For example, a nonrunner may find a one-mile jog utterly daunting. But with practice, over time, that same person may find himself or herself gliding along with relative ease on a five-mile run. The unattainable often becomes attainable with practice. It is the same with reading music. At first a sheet of music may appear to be nothing more than an unintelligible series of bizarre glyphs. But by becoming familiar with those symbols one can eventually "hear" the music on the page. Or consider meditation. At first, meditating can be a frustrating experience during which the mind seems to be filled with buzzing bees. Quiescence is a laughable fantasy. But over time, one can learn to calm the thought process, and meditation becomes a dip into a clear, pellucid pool of pure mind. It takes practice.

The human energy system works in two directions. On the one hand, it is the system through which life energy and intelligence animate and sustain us. On the other hand, it is a route to vast dimensions of energy and intelligence far beyond our bodily needs and our intellectual comprehension, a sort of highway to the infinite. You can play within the human energy system, getting familiar with it to the point that you can tap your mind and your senses into the energy current that flows through it. Over time you can become adept at following that flow beyond the body/mind. I like to refer to this as "surfing the current." However one chooses to describe it, this is the pursuit of sages and yogis and mystics throughout all history.

If you only read and talk about the human energy system, it will remain just an ephemeral abstraction. But by practicing the methods described in this book, the human energy system can become real to you through your own experience. You will then have the opportunity to explore the breadth and depth of the intelligent life force that flows within you.

3 THE CHAKRAS

As mentioned in the previous chapter, inherent within the human energy system are the chakras, concentrated vortices of energy. While there are many distinct places throughout the body/mind where concentrated energy resides, such as at the various acupuncture points, the seven chakras are the primary energetic centers, the major nexuses of energy distribution for the rest of the human energy system. Located along the spinal pathway, each chakra is associated with particular organs, glands, and nerve plexuses. Each chakra is also associated with certain states of consciousness.

The seven chakras function in concert, as do the organs, glands, nerves, and other systems of the body. Like these physical aspects, the chakras may be weak or strong, balanced or imbalanced. Just as massage can soothe an aching muscle or the right nutrient can stimulate a gland to function well, the chakras are influenced by methods of power like the Five Tibetans. The purpose of practicing the Five Tibetans is to influence the chakras so they can function at peak activity and condition, in balance and harmony with each other. And what is the reason to pursue peak chakra functioning? When the human energy system is working well, then the body and mind are healthy, vital, and balanced. To attend to the chakras is not a diversion into some ephemeral realm of vague mystical mumbo-jumbo. The function of the chakras affects every aspect of who we are and how we experience life.

THREE PRIMARY ENERGETIC PATHWAYS

The seven chakras lie along the spinal column and are connected by three major energetic pathways known as *ida*, *pingala*, and *sushumna*. While I typically eschew Sanskrit names simply because almost nobody is fluent in that ancient language, these are the only names I know for the three pathways, so let the Sanskrit stand. The channels run from the base of the spine to the top of the head, conveying energy from one chakra to another. Sushumna, the central channel, is the energetic counterpart to the spinal cord and is the core channel of all energetic flow in the human energy system. Sushumna is the primary pathway through which energy flows from the base of the spine to the top of the head. Kundalini energy travels through the sushumna, illuminating body and mind. (Kundalini energy will be discussed in the next chapter.)

The origins of sushumna and the other primary energetic channels, ida and pingala, are at the base of the spine, the location of the first chakra. Ida runs up the left side of the central channel; pingala ascends the right side. These two channels travel upward, intertwining with each other at each chakra. Their physical counterparts are the ganglionic nerve chains that run alongside the spinal cord. Ida is connected to the left nostril, and pingala is connected to the right. Ida is considered lunar in nature, while pingala is regarded as solar. It's interesting to note that the caduceus, the insignia of physicians, is a representation of these three major energetic pathways. Depicted as a staff with two serpents winding around it and a pair of wings on top, the caduceus symbolizes the ascent of consciousness from lower chakras to higher ones. The wings of the caduceus represent the two-petaled third eye, the wisdom eye or eye of revelation.

The Five Tibetans help to balance the lunar and solar forces of ida and pingala, and assist in channeling a steady, concentrated flow of energy through sushumna, the central channel. Each exercise physically stimulates various nerve plexuses and glands that lie along the spinal pathway, as well as the spine itself and the ganglionic nerve chains. Enhanced energetic activity in the spinal nerves and primary energetic pathways results from the physical pressure and nerve stimulation that occur during practice of the Five Tibetans. Over time, an energetic charge builds up in the body/mind. Not only do the Five Tibetans become easier to practice, but the energetic effect they produce is greatly amplified. Energy flows more smoothly through the central channel, owing to a gradual elimination of obstructions. As this process occurs, physical health and vitality improve, the mind becomes more powerful, and one can enter into high states of meditation with increasingly greater ease.

THE SEVEN CHAKRAS

The First Chakra

The first chakra is located at the base of the spine at the perineum, the spot between the anus and the genitals. The energy flowing through this center is dense, vital, and powerful. This chakra is associated with the most basic aspects of human survival. Survival is a drive imprinted into our genetic makeup. It is the root of our consciousness. The most ancient part of the human brain, the reptilian inner brain, functions mainly in support of survival. The first chakra influences the system in the same ways as the reptilian brain.

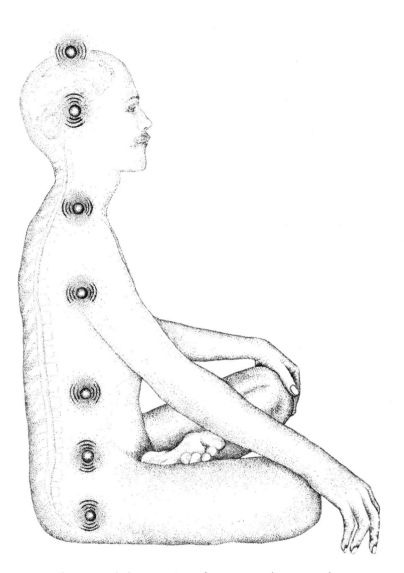

The seven chakras, vortices of concentrated power within the human energy system.

Just as the first chakra is at the root of the spine, so the influence of this chakra is at the root of all consciousness.

> **Primary functions of the first chakra:** survival, power, the promotion of vital life energy, elimination
> **Associated organs:** large intestine and rectum
> **Associated glands:** adrenal glands
> **Major related nerve center:** coccygeal and sacral plexuses
> **Sanskrit name:** *muladhara*

The Second Chakra

Located at the point of the spine close to the reproductive organs, the second chakra is fundamentally associated with creativity. Creativity is made manifest in many ways and underlies many activities. As the most fundamental act of human creativity is procreation, the second chakra is the center of sexual energy, of procreation and regeneration. Sexual energy underlies every act of individual expression. It is a creative force, the influence of which extends far beyond sexual activity to include thought, feeling, behavior, dress. Sexual energy informs art, music, fashion, even architecture and automotive design. It is an all-pervading force.

Sexual orgasm is both an experience of biological satisfaction and a transcendent experience. Sexual orgasm is so highly sought after because during orgasm one experiences, however briefly, a sense of timelessness. This same timeless rapture is common to mystical states and is fundamental to successful shamanistic rituals. The second chakra is a highly active center, the energy of which permeates virtually everything we do. It is fundamental to both basic creativity and higher ecstasy.

> **Primary functions of the second chakra:** creativity, procreation, sexual function, the promotion of vitality

Associated organs: large intestine, bladder, kidneys, and
   reproductive organs
Associated glands: reproductive glands
Major related nerve center: prostatic plexus (male) and
   utero-vaginal plexus (female)
Sanskrit name: *svadhisthana*

The Third Chakra

The third chakra, located at the solar plexus, is the center of the
individual self. Individuation of consciousness develops beyond
basic survival and continuation of the species to a sense of oneself as
a unique being. The third chakra is the vortex for the individuation
of consciousness. It is the center of personal power and the origin of
will. The third chakra generates the drive toward self-assertion, personal determination, and individual strength, preparing us to meet
the challenges of living in the world. This center can be enormously
powerful and is associated with personal charisma.

Primary functions of the third chakra: will, personal
   power, digestion, and assimilation of nutrients
Associated organs: liver, spleen, stomach, and small
   intestine
Associated gland: pancreas
Major related nerve center: solar plexus
Sanskrit name: *manipura*

The Fourth Chakra

The fourth chakra lies at the point of the spine across from the
sternum, at the center of the chest, and is considered to be the
focal point of love and compassion in the human energy system.
It is at the fourth chakra that human consciousness moves beyond
self-centeredness into an expanded awareness of connection with

the rest of the world. Lying midway between the lower three chakras and the higher three centers, the fourth chakra marks the point of conscious departure from lower to higher awareness. The energy that flows from this center is directed beyond personal survival to consideration of others. To gain access to the higher functions of creativity and awareness, one must consciously "pass through" the fourth chakra.

> **Primary functions of the fourth chakra:** love; compassion; immunity; heart, lung, and bronchial functions
> **Associated organs:** heart and lungs
> **Associated gland:** thymus
> **Major related nerve center:** cardiac plexus
> **Sanskrit name:** *anahata*

The Fifth Chakra

The fifth chakra is located at the spine directly behind the center of the throat. Through this chakra flow the energies for the higher functions of communication, creativity, and personal expression. The power of this chakra is most noticeable in the activity of speaking, which may well be the most influential of all human behaviors. When this chakra is well developed one can speak with tremendous force and persuasiveness. All creative activity involves a process by which we express something from deep within. When the fifth chakra is strong, such expression can be dramatic, powerful, and deeply moving. This chakra is so potent that its force can be spellbinding.

> **Primary functions of the fifth chakra:** higher creativity and communication
> **Associated organs:** vocal chords
> **Associated gland:** thyroid

Major related nerve center: pharyngeal plexus
Sanskrit name: *visuddha*

The Sixth Chakra

The sixth chakra resides directly behind the root of the nose, between the eyebrows and inward toward the center of the head. Also known as the third eye or wisdom eye, this chakra is the location of higher intelligence and supranormal vision. The third eye is the center of insight, an inner vision directed by wisdom and a deep understanding of the subtle forces at play in any situation. When the third eye is "open" one can clearly see the past, present, and future. Individuals with this extraordinary vision are the few true clairvoyants. The higher intelligence associated with the sixth chakra is expansive and sensitive. An open third eye enables one to easily achieve desired outcomes that are positive and generative.

Primary functions of the sixth chakra: higher intelligence, clairvoyance, insight, refined hearing
Associated organ: brain
Associated gland: pituitary
Major related nerve center: cavernous plexus
Sanskrit name: *ajna*

The Seventh Chakra

Located at the crown of the head, the seventh chakra is the center of cosmic consciousness, a state of absolute awareness and integration with the primary creative force of the universe. It is an unconditional state of total fulfillment, the embodiment of total freedom, wisdom, energy, insight, and joy. Upon awakening the seventh chakra, one finds that cosmic consciousness is the natural human condition. Such awakening is usually the product of intense purification, inner refinement, and spiritual work; however, since cosmic consciousness, or illumination, or enlightenment, cannot be known by the intellect, one cannot say that there are only prescribed ways to attain this condition. The truth is, genuine illumination is outside the scope of intellectual thought. It can only be known through direct experience.

Primary function of the seventh chakra: cosmic consciousness
Associated organ: brain
Associated gland: pineal gland
Major related nerve center: cavernous plexus
Sanskrit name: *sahasrara*

CHAKRA PSYCHOLOGY

The chakras exist within the human energy system, creating in each individual a unique balance of a broad range of influences, from survival instincts to vastly expanded awareness. The chakras can therefore also be used as a model to consider one's own mind. By reflecting upon the nature of our own thoughts, inclinations, perceptions, desires, and actions, we can fairly accurately identify which chakras are dominant within us. We can also determine ways we might develop in order to be more fully expressive of the latent forces within us.

For example, a person who is consumed by personal ambition and takes every opportunity to get ahead in a way that furthers his or her own personal fortune, while focusing on little else, is strongly influenced by the third chakra. Having a strong third chakra is by no means a bad thing. Doing for oneself is good and valuable. But it can be terribly limiting if there are no other strong influences. For such a person, performing service for others is a terrific way of achieving a more balanced mentality and chakra influence. There is nothing mystical or esoteric about it. If you're self-consumed, then doing something for others is a way of retraining your attention and energy. By contrast, a person who devotes himself or herself largely to the comfort and well-being of others is very likely a fourth-chakra "type," a giver and lover of humanity.

A person who is dominated by influences from the lower chakras can simultaneously be influenced by the higher centers as well. There are many power-mad gurus and sages who have paranormal perceptions and occult abilities that indicate some higher-chakra activity, but who operate from a fundamentally low-chakra base, using their powers to cheat, deceive, and dominate others. Don't be fooled: psychic abilities do not indicate a fundamentally integrated person who works from a higher chakra level. It is important not to be awestruck when someone demonstrates psychic abilities. Consider the whole person. Or as the Zen saying goes, "Look to the obvious." If the person with psychic abilities is also loving, kind, charitable, and quick to serve others with little or no concern for personal gain, then he or she may in fact be well integrated. Take time to find out. Don't assume that just because someone wears a turban, speaks with an exotic vocal lilt, and spews mantras at the drop of a dollar, he or she is either well integrated or interested in your well-being. Spiritual hucksters are everywhere.

Chakra psychology is a valuable tool for greater self-understanding. If we can honestly assess the influences within us, we can then work on those areas in which we may be lacking or consciously modify influences so extreme that they work to our detriment. If you toil ceaselessly for the benefit of others (a fourth-chakra type) to the point that you put yourself at great peril by utterly neglecting your own basic needs, then you may need to work on your survival instincts. After all, if you really want to serve others to the best possible extent, you need to be alive and well. Otherwise, your mission to serve will be short-lived. If you want to live a balanced life but find that you are so sex-crazed (a very strong second-chakra influence) that you spend most of your time attempting to satisfy insatiable sexual urges, you may need to practice moving beyond self-gratification by involving yourself in some form of service or community work. Some people, sometimes referred to as "bliss ninnies," are lost in a little etheric world of their own (a likely third-eye dominance) and lack any sense of grounded-ness. Physical labor is very helpful with this kind of chakra imbalance, as is challenging intellectual work.

The instructions for chakra meditation in chapter 9 are of great benefit in balancing the energies of the chakras. But meditation alone is insufficient. In addition, self-analysis is of great value, and action is critical. If, for example, you wish to be less spaced-out and in the clouds, then performing a chakra meditation is helpful. But that meditation needs to be supplemented by specific physical and mental activities that challenge you and demand your full mental attention and physical participation. If you are excessively self-absorbed and hyperambitious and wish to be more outer-directed, then meditation will help. But consciously engaging in some form of work for others will help you make substantive changes. In other words, chakra meditation isn't a mystical quick fix for personal imbalance. It simply helps, along with a great deal of critical self-examination and action.

The variations of chakra imbalance are endless, and virtually everybody is imbalanced in some ways. Chakra influences permeate the entire body and mind, and can be overwhelming because they work at every level of who we are. It often takes extraordinary effort to achieve a greater measure of balance. Furthermore, it is extremely difficult to assess ourselves honestly, because we humans are endowed with extraordinary powers of self-deception. Thus the task of creating balance is rarely a simple one. It is a struggle that demands strength of character, tremendous vitality, trust in greater awareness, and the kind of clear mind that comes from meditation practice. Nonetheless, an examination of the chakras, coupled with the most frank self-assessment that we can muster, can be an illuminating step on the road to personal balance and harmony.

4 KUNDALINI

In the entire realm of yoga, nothing is more misunderstood, sought after, maligned, reviled, worshiped, feared, and misrepresented than kundalini, the primordial energy that enlivens us and is, as Gopi Krishna calls it, "the seat of all genius."

The human energy system is the circuitry through which life energy flows within us. This energy is called by many names, including chi, ki, bio-energy, and the force. The terminology varies depending upon culture, tradition, the lineage of teachers, and language, but the energetic force remains the same. I choose to refer to the life energy as kundalini, because the yogic articulation of this force seems more accurate and complete than any other I have ever found.

The word *kundalini* invokes curiosity, fear, and suspicion. It is misunderstood largely because sensational literature has portrayed the most lurid, outlandish aspects of this force while minimizing the benign fundamentals. Kundalini is the primary life force within us, the primary evolutionary force, a sliver of the Absolute dwelling within the human body. Kundalini is sometimes referred to as the serpent power, portrayed as a snake coiled at the base of the spine.

In fact, kundalini is a force within the human brain that activates the chakras; it is typically first *felt* at the base of the spine, in the first chakra. The *Siva Samhita* describes this when Siva says, "From the base or root of the palate, the sushumna extends downwards, till it reaches the Muladhara (first chakra) and the perineum . . ." (verse 121), and then in verse 124, "In that hole of the sushumna there dwells as its inner force the kundalini." Kundalini is not a mystical snake; it is the primary psychobiological force. Kundalini is the energy that enlivens, vivifies, and motivates the body and mind.

Kundalini is always active. It fuels the entire human energy system, causing life energy to circulate within us on a continual basis. For most people, the extent of kundalini activity is minimal, though it is always operating within us to some extent. If you could compare kundalini to running water, most people have a small garden sprinkler running at low flow within them, while the full force of kundalini is equal to the immense power of Niagara Falls. The full potential of kundalini is massive, inconceivable.

The practice of yoga strengthens the channels of the human energy system and prepares the body for enhanced kundalini flow. Meditation activates greater kundalini activity, increasing the intensity of this force. As the body and energy channels are better prepared through yoga practice, a person can withstand more kundalini activity. As the mind becomes more focused and concentrated in its attention, more energy gets moving. This in a nutshell is how it works.

The arousal of kundalini energy can happen in many ways. It can occur slowly, almost imperceptibly over time, producing a steady but gradual increase in energy and mental alertness. Or it can occur in stages during which you may experience phenomena such as sensations of warm energetic currents rising up the spine. These sensations are relatively common among people who practice yoga and meditation. But kundalini can also arise suddenly and without warning, and its intensity may be incapacitating. Kundalini energy can burst up the spine like a bolt of lightning with intense heat, blasting open the chakras like dynamite exploding mud out the mouth of a cave. Experiences of this kind can be scary and disorienting, and are responsible for the lurid and ominous tales told of kundalini. If you practice yoga and meditate with concentration, you will be reasonably well prepared to accept an increase of kundalini flow within you. I say reasonably well prepared because you cannot be fully ready to receive something as monumental as the power of kundalini. It can surprise and overwhelm the strongest and best-trained people. The only thing you can do when kundalini moves powerfully through you is surrender to the experience. Do not fight it. Kundalini is stronger than anything you have ever encountered.

The arousal of kundalini is a process that has plenty of latitude to it. In other words, you can set a course to more fully awaken the kundalini energy, but you cannot manage every aspect of how and when that will occur. As the primary psychobiological force, kundalini is something that almost everyone has experienced, usually during moments of sudden inspiration or within orgasm. The experience of falling into space, of losing control and feeling a wave of ecstasy upon orgasm, is a sexual kundalini experience. At moments of profound reverie, when the world seems particularly magnificent and rich, kundalini is at play.

With training you can increase your capacity for kundalini flow and stimulate more of that force within you. You can safely accomplish this through practice of the Five Tibetans and the meditation techniques in chapter 9. The chakras and the primary energy pathways will become increasingly activated and vital, opening up a little more each day as increased kundalini energy circulates through you. The urge to practice yoga or to meditate comes from kundalini. It is this force that impels us forward, encouraging us to become involved in pursuits that purify the body and enhance the mind. Many changes occur as the flow of kundalini increases. You feel stronger and more alert, and your sensory acuity is enhanced. I have found that my senses are more finely honed now than when I was younger. The senses are chakra related, and everything is enhanced when kundalini is stronger within the body. Food becomes more flavorful, subtle aromas are easier to smell, colors appear more vivid, touch becomes more sensitive, music has more acoustic dimension, and so on. The world becomes a more vital, sensual place.

With greater kundalini flow your basic energy level also increases. Some people initially require more rest than usual when they first undertake a yoga practice because they are experiencing major physical and energetic changes. Eventually, less rest will be required daily. You will find yourself more active and stimulated, sleeping less and maintaining a more constant level of energy throughout the day. You will find that you can apply yourself to challenging mental tasks for long periods of time with less fatigue. In addition, you might find that you can simply will yourself to be more energetic when it is really needed.

Sleep patterns also change with increased kundalini flow. In addition to possibly requiring less sleep, your dreams may become unusually vivid or even prophetic. Meditation practice can open you to experience lucid dreaming, a state in which you are consciously aware, during sleep, that what is taking place is a dream.

There are some classic somatic experiences that often accompany kundalini movement, the most common of which is a sensation of warmth at the base of the spine. This feeling can be quite pleasurable; it may at times feel as though you are sitting on something hot. Often this experience is accompanied by particularly strong sexual urges.

One frequent experience I had during my early days of kundalini practice was spinal vibration. For a while, every time I sat to meditate my spine would quiver slightly and at a high speed, as though it were a vibrator. This was not due to muscle fatigue or strain, and only occurred during meditation. Eventually it stopped altogether.

One of the most exciting kundalini experiences is when a sudden burst of energy shoots up the spine, often accompanied by a sensation of heat and occasionally by vivid colors as well. It's an inner light show of sorts. One usually experiences a sense of joy, expansion, and equanimity. It is a lovely thing. When this happens it is a time to focus your attention, to meditate and make more of the situation than just a fleeting experience. By doing so, you may be able to mentally tap into the kundalini power in a way that will create lasting effects in terms of feeling clear minded, vividly alert, strong, and enthusiastic about life. Though most kundalini experiences are short-lived, sometimes they can go on for a long time. I once experienced a six-week period of heightened kundalini activity. During that time I ate moderately, slept very little, did a great deal of yoga, meditated a lot, and was in a continual state of ecstasy.

In his book *The Kundalini Experience*, Dr. Lee Sannella says that "The kundalini process, like deep meditation, stirs up the sediments of the unconscious and confronts a person with just those psychic materials he or she wishes to inspect least of all." The idea that kundalini arousal will stir up mental muck is true. You may find as you get involved with kundalini meditation that things come up in your mind that are decidedly not pleasant. When this occurs, try to keep from being attached to the phenomena that arise. Instead, let the energy within you steadily increase, and let unpleasant thoughts, feelings, and sensations pass away as if blown by the wind. This is what the Hindus refer to as burning up old karma, accumulated psychic dross that you may have dragged around with you for many lifetimes. There is no way to go through a true awakening of kundalini without going through a mental quagmire. This is because we all have fears, distortions, perversions, and deeply buried mental convolutions that we must work through. Kundalini stirs these things up because it is an expression of pure consciousness and energy. It is like a strong light illuminating a dark cave. If there are bat droppings and old bones in the cave, they will come to light. Everybody has some mental muck to get rid of, and when kundalini activity increases, you will be confronted by yours.

Kundalini is nothing less than the primary force of life within us. The extent to which kundalini manifests within a person is partly due to effort. If you practice the Five Tibetans and engage in the kundalini meditation described in chapter 9, there is an excellent likelihood that you will begin to arouse the largely dormant kundalini energy within, awakening yourself to a new, brilliant world of experience and awareness.

5 BREATHING

Breath is fundamental to human life. Breathing is a simple, automatic function. We breathe from the moment we are born, and when we stop breathing, we die. It's very simple. We humans are very versatile and adaptable. We can go for long periods of time without food, as evidenced by the great fasting heroics of Gandhi and others. We can go without water for a few days. We can go without pizza, movies, a ride in a car, or even sex for greatly extended periods. The monks of Mt. Hiei in Japan (who are known as "running monks" because they run as much as fifty-two miles per day) endure an ordeal during which they go without food, water, or sleep for nine days. This they refer to as an "ultimate fast." (Do not try this at home!) The point is, we can go for some time without many things, some of them essential to life. If, however, you go without breathing for a relatively short period of time, you will be released from your mortal form.

Breathing is the most primary of all forms of nourishment. When we breathe we take in a mixture of gasses, especially oxygen, which is needed to feed our cells. We also take in a subtle form of energy called *prana*. Just as oxygen feeds the cells of our bodies, so prana feeds the human energy system, the energetic substrate of the human body. Though breathing is a simple and natural function, it can be adjusted and modified to yield particular results. Prana from the breath can be channeled to build, purify, and strengthen the entire human energy system. Thus virtually every system of body/mind development, from all systems of yoga to the multitudinous forms of martial arts, employs methods of breath control. It is said in some yoga scriptures that when you master the breath, you master your destiny. This may be a bit of an overstatement, but it *is* true that when you master the breath you gain tremendous control over your body and mind.

In this chapter I describe proper breathing so you can get your practice of the Five Tibetans off to a good start. Please be sure to practice breathing carefully, according to the instructions given here. Sometimes people feel that they should practice more of something at the onset, starting out with great intensity and doing more than is recommended. That is not a wise approach to take with breathing exercises. If you feel the need to be intense then do five hundred sit-ups, run ten miles, and tire yourself out. But do not overdo breathing practice. Simple, basic breathing methods can be extremely powerful. Because breathing is something natural that we do all the time, it may seem that strenuous practice of breathing exercises would cause no negative consequences, but this is not the case. You can harm yourself by overdoing breathing exercises. The best way to progress well in breathing practice and yoga is to learn carefully and continue to practice with increasingly greater care and precision as time goes on.

As you engage in *pranayam*, the science of breath control, a number of changes occur. Your body begins to detoxify, expelling poisons from the liver, kidneys, bowels, and skin. Initially you may feel lightheaded during pranayam, due in part to the greatly increased amount of oxygen going to your brain. This sensation of lightness is not only due to oxygen intake. As you practice controlled breathing, you break through obstructions in the human energy system. Blockages along the energetic pathways or within the chakras are dissolved with consistent breathing practice. As the human energy system conducts increasing power, you will feel lighter. Sometimes it will feel as though every cell in the whole body is dancing in light.

This in fact is the case, reasonable when you consider that all of the known universe is energy and light. Matter is not really solid, but is instead a heavy, condensed form of energy. Each atomic particle of your being is suspended in space and is dancing around other atomic particles at a rapid rate. Becoming "lighter" is not a matter of simply being less heavy but of actually assimilating more light into yourself. Through consistent breathing practice and meditation, you draw more pure, clear, white light into your energy system, literally lighting up the chakras.

Breathing is a complete yoga unto itself, and there are hundreds of variations to the practice of pranayam. Since the focus of this book is the Five Tibetans and not a full exploration of all aspects of yoga, we will focus on three breathing methods only. The first is the normal breath; the second is the long, deep breath; and the third is a breath that is performed after each of the Five Tibetans. **Practice breathing on an empty stomach** to avoid nausea and cramping, and to allow the energy to circulate as freely as possible throughout your system.

THE NORMAL BREATH

Sit in a comfortable position, either cross-legged or in a straight-backed chair. Keep your spine erect, sitting as tall and well aligned as possible. Relax your shoulders and chest. Place one hand with the palm on your abdomen so you can easily feel what is happening during the exercise. Placing your hand on your abdomen will not be necessary once you are familiar with this manner of breathing. Take a light breath through the nose, letting your abdomen fill and expand outward with the breath. Exhale through either the nose or mouth, relaxing the belly. During this exercise your chest should not move at all. This breath is much like filling a balloon—as you inhale through your nose, your abdomen expands. As you exhale through the nose or mouth, your abdomen collapses. As simple as this sounds, it is very important to beginning breath practice, so go over this exercise repeatedly. Practice easy, gentle breathing for about two minutes, expanding the abdomen as you inhale through the nose and letting the abdomen collapse as you gently exhale through the nose or mouth.

This is the manner of relaxed breathing that you should maintain throughout the day. From this practice you may find that you have been breathing in a different way, sucking in your abdomen upon inhaling. This is altogether too common, and it may feel strange to reverse your habitual breathing style. Do persevere. Though it takes practice and concentration to retrain yourself to breathe properly, the benefits of normal, full-belly breathing are enormous.

Please note that it is important to inhale through your nose whenever possible. Inhaling through the mouth bypasses breath-regulating mechanisms and can cause dizziness, nervousness, and other physical and emotional problems. Be sure to inhale regularly through the nose. Exhalation may be either through the nose or mouth.

THE LONG, DEEP BREATH

This is similar to the normal breath except that it is deeper. To practice this breath, sit in a comfortable position and place one hand with the palm flat on your abdomen and one at the center of your chest. The hand placement is for learning this breath, not for regular practice. As you inhale, draw the breath in through the nose, filling your abdomen as in the normal breath, but this time continue inhaling until your lungs are also full to the top and your chest is expanded. Then gently exhale through either the nose or mouth.

It is important that you work with this breath until you can perform it correctly and with ease. The long, deep breath is much like filling a glass of water—as you pour water in from the top, the glass fills from the bottom up. It is the same with the breath—it comes in from the top of your body but it fills you up from the lower abdomen first, eventually filling the chest cavity as well. Practice this breath for several minutes every day until it comes easily and automatically.

Any time you need to relieve stress (except after a large meal), sit comfortably and breathe deeply and slowly, drawing the breath way down inside you and then letting it go easily and evenly. Doing this literally washes away tension and will leave you feeling calm, relaxed, and invigorated.

THE INTERIM BREATH

This breath is performed two times only, after each of the Five Tibetans. Take a few minutes to practice this, as it is an important part of the practice of these exercises.

Stand straight with your feet together and your hands on your hips. Take a long, full, deep breath, inhaling through the nose. Exhale through the mouth with your lips pursed in an "O" (see figure 2 on page 40).

Now that you have practiced breathing you are ready to learn the Five Tibetans.

6 THE FIVE TIBETANS

Here, after much introduction, are the Five Tibetans. The Five Tibetans stimulate full energy flow through the chakras and enliven corresponding nerves, organs, and glands. These exercises also tone and strengthen the major muscle groups, contributing to a strong, resilient physique. Once you are familiar with the exercises, practice of the Five Tibetans will take about five or six minutes daily.

The Five Tibetans are ideally practiced twenty-one times each. Oddly enough, there is no need to exceed twenty-one repetitions, as the desired energetic effect of the Five Tibetans is achieved at that number. I know of no harm from performing a greater number, but it simply isn't necessary. Most people need to work up to that number of repetitions, so don't be concerned if it is difficult to practice the full complement from the start. It takes nearly every beginner a month or longer to work up to the full twenty-one repetitions.

In the beginning, start out with ten or twelve repetitions of each exercise. Build your practice at your own pace. You will be doing yourself a great deal of good by practicing any number, and there is a lot of satisfaction to be gained from working your way up to twenty-one times each. Take your time, practicing daily and with as much precision as possible. Even as you are building up to twenty-one repetitions of each exercise, you will start to feel stronger and more energetic.

To ensure that you are practicing properly, carefully read the instructions for each exercise, and refer to the accompanying photographs. The Five Tibetans are represented accurately here, so you can model your posture, footing, and overall position according to what you see on these pages.

TIBETAN #1

⊕

Stand up straight with your arms outstretched to the sides (figure 1). Fingers are together; palms are open and facing downward. Holding this arm position, spin full circle in a clockwise direction. (If you were to turn your head to the right, that is the direction in which you want to spin.) Repeat the spin twenty-one times without a break.

When you finish spinning, stand with your feet together and your hands on your hips (figure 2). Take a full, deep breath, inhaling through the nose. Exhale through the mouth with your lips pursed in an "O." Repeat the inhale and exhale, completing two full breaths before moving on to Tibetan #2.

You may experience some dizziness when you first practice this exercise. Be careful, and don't push it. This exercise strengthens the vestibular apparatus, the balance mechanism residing in the inner ear. With regular practice the dizziness will stop and the spin will become easy and fluid, even at very fast speeds. This is the same motion practiced by Islamic Dervishes, Sufi mystics who twirl at rapid speeds for long periods of time. These mystics are known as "whirling Dervishes."

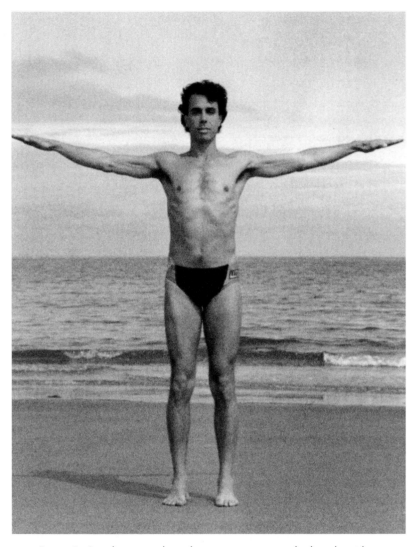

Figure 1. Stand up straight with your arms outstretched to the sides. Fingers are together; palms are open and facing downward. Holding this arm position, spin full circle in a clockwise direction. (If you were to turn your head to the right, that is the direction in which you want to spin.) Repeat the spin twenty-one times without a break.

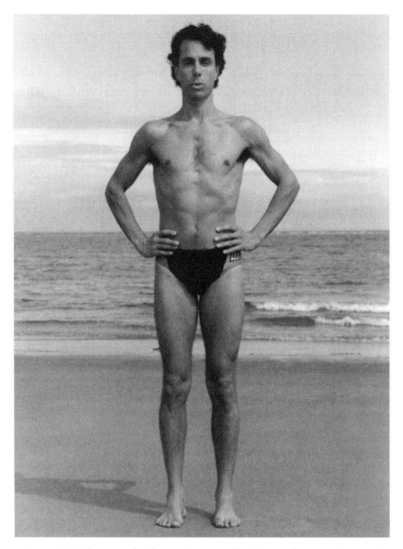

Figure 2. When you finish spinning, stand with your feet together and your hands on your hips. Take a full, deep breath, inhaling through the nose. Exhale through the mouth with your lips pursed in an "O." Repeat the inhale and exhale, completing two full breaths before moving on to Tibetan #2.

TIBETAN #2

⊕

Lie on your back on a mat or rug. Your legs are fully extended, ankles flexed and touching. Arms are by your sides with the palms flat on the floor (figure 3). Inhale through the nose, lift your legs a little past a ninety-degree angle, and raise your head, tucking your chin into your chest (figure 4). This is all done in one smooth motion. Your toes point toward the sky; your lower back should remain flat on the ground.

Exhale through either your nose or mouth, bringing your legs and head down to the starting position—completely flat on the ground. Repeat the entire motion twenty-one times, inhaling as you raise your legs and head, exhaling as you bring them down.

When you are finished, stand with your feet together and hands on hips (figure 2). Take two full, deep breaths, inhaling through the nose and exhaling through the mouth, with your lips pursed in an "O."

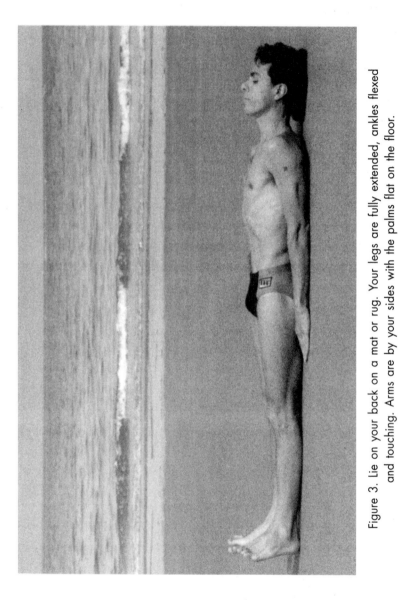

Figure 3. Lie on your back on a mat or rug. Your legs are fully extended, ankles flexed and touching. Arms are by your sides with the palms flat on the floor.

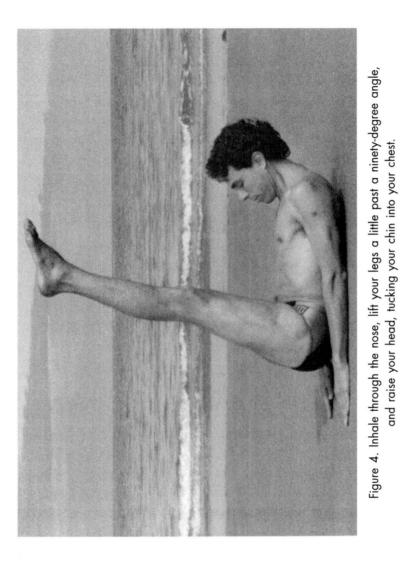

Figure 4. Inhale through the nose, lift your legs a little past a ninety-degree angle, and raise your head, tucking your chin into your chest.

TIBETAN #3

⊕

Kneel with the balls of your feet resting on the ground. Your knees are about four inches apart. Place your palms against the backs of your thighs just below the buttocks. Your spine is erect, with your chin tucked into your chest (figure 5).

Inhale through the nose, arching back from the waist. Drop your head as far back as you comfortably can (figure 6). Your hands will support you as you lean back. Then exhale through either the nose or mouth, as you return to the starting position. Repeat the entire motion twenty-one times in a steady, unbroken rhythm.

When you finish, stand with your feet together and your hands on your hips (figure 2). Take two full, deep breaths, inhaling through the nose and exhaling through the mouth, with your lips pursed in an "O."

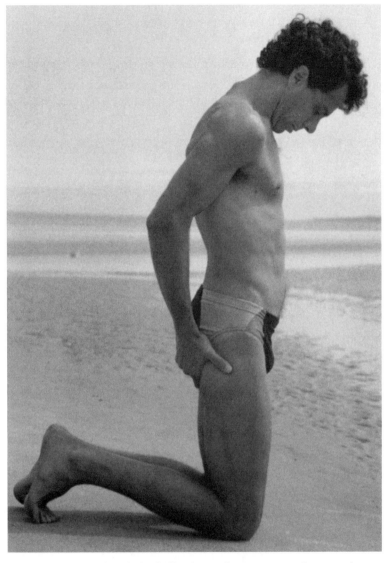

Figure 5. Kneel with the balls of your feet resting on the ground.
Your knees are about four inches apart. Place your palms against
the backs of your thighs just below the buttocks. Your spine is erect,
with your chin tucked into your chest.

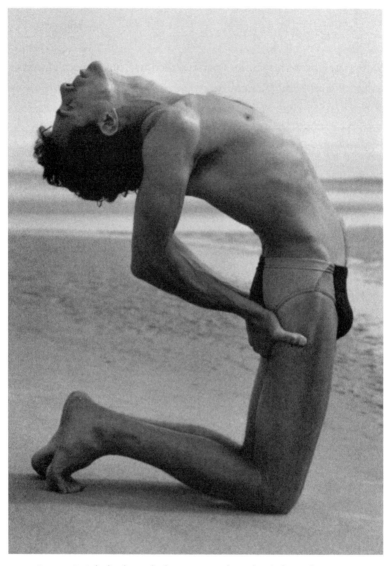

Figure 6. Inhale through the nose, arching back from the waist.
Drop your head as far back as you comfortably can.

TIBETAN #4

⊕

Sit up straight with your legs outstretched in front of you. Place the palms of your hands flat on the ground beside your hips. Positioning of the hands is very important; they must be placed exactly alongside the hips. Tuck your chin into your chest (figure 7).

Inhaling through the nose, raise your hips as you bend your knees, bringing the soles of your feet flat to the ground and dropping your head all the way back (figure 8). You will come into a position in which the trunk is parallel to the ground while the arms and legs are perpendicular. Exhale through either the nose or mouth as you come down to the starting position. Repeat this motion twenty-one times in a steady, unbroken rhythm. Do not let your feet slide. The feet should stay in the same place through this whole exercise. Also, the arms should not bend; the movement is instead accomplished by pivoting at the shoulders.

Stand when you are finished, feet together and hands on hips (figure 2). Take two full, deep breaths, inhaling through the nose and exhaling through the mouth, with your lips pursed in an "O."

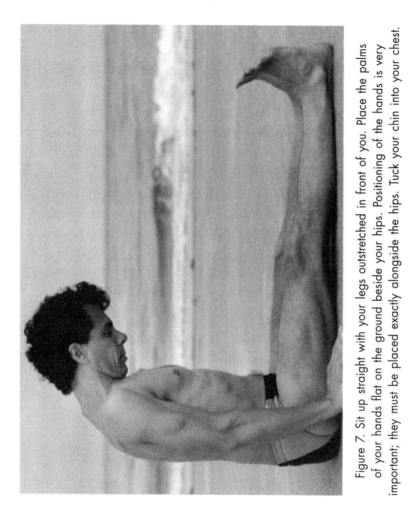

Figure 7. Sit up straight with your legs outstretched in front of you. Place the palms of your hands flat on the ground beside your hips. Positioning of the hands is very important; they must be placed exactly alongside the hips. Tuck your chin into your chest.

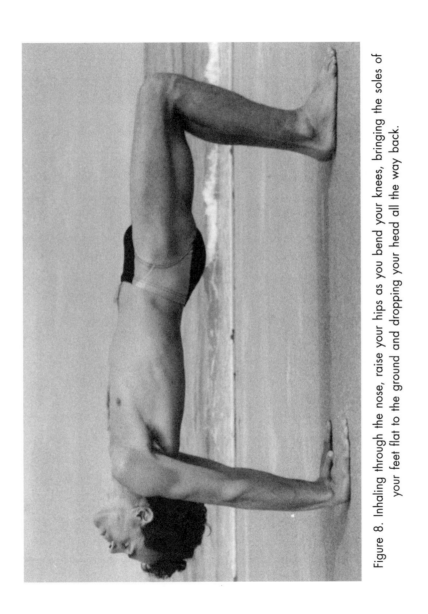

Figure 8. Inhaling through the nose, raise your hips as you bend your knees, bringing the soles of your feet flat to the ground and dropping your head all the way back.

TIBETAN #5

⊕

Begin this exercise by supporting yourself on the palms of your hands and the balls of your feet. Both the arms and the legs are about two feet apart. Your head is up and back (figure 9). Keeping your arms and legs straight, inhale through the nose as you raise your buttocks and tuck your chin into your chest, bringing your body up into a perfect triangle (figure 10). Exhale through either your nose or mouth as you swing back down to the starting position. Except for the palms of your hands and the balls of your feet, your body remains off the ground during the entirety of this exercise, and your arms and legs do not bend at all. Repeat the entire motion twenty-one times in a smooth, unbroken rhythm.

Upon finishing, stand with your feet together and hands on hips (figure 2). Take two full, deep breaths, inhaling through the nose and exhaling through the mouth, with your lips pursed in an "O."

⊕

When you have finished performing all five exercises, lie down on your back and relax for several minutes. Let the breath be gentle and easy. Notice any new sensations in your body.

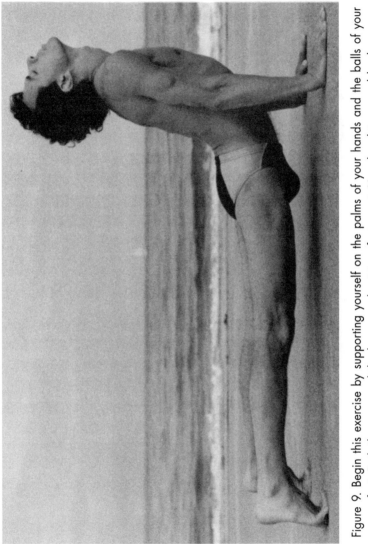

Figure 9. Begin this exercise by supporting yourself on the palms of your hands and the balls of your feet. Both the arms and the legs are about two feet apart. Your head is up and back.

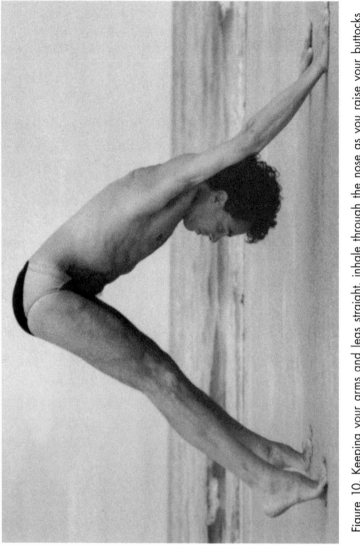

Figure 10. Keeping your arms and legs straight, inhale through the nose as you raise your buttocks and tuck your chin into your chest, bringing your body up into a perfect triangle.

AN ACCOMPANIMENT TO
THE FIVE TIBETANS
⊕

According to Peter Kelder's account, the Five Tibetans originated in a monastic community whose members were celibate. Celibacy is standard for monastic societies—at least, that's the classic rule. The reality is that in many monastic communities, whether Hindu, Catholic, Muslim, or Buddhist, plenty of illicit sexual activity takes place. This happens because all beings are sexual beings. For many people, celibacy is an unendurable exercise in frustration.

Many religions and spiritual traditions regard sexual activity as a distraction from "higher" pursuits, arguing that fulfilling the appetites of the flesh equals neglecting the aspirations of the soul. Thus monks and nuns are typically required to live without sex. It is well documented that this deprivation leads to clandestine liaisons. Nuns get at each other; priests get at each other; monks get at each other; priests, monks, and nuns get at neophytes, and so on. Human beings simply weren't meant to live without physical intimacy. If sex can't be open and free, then it will be clandestine and distorted.

Beyond the belief that sex is a spiritual distraction (I regard it as a powerful spiritual tool), some traditions teach that the loss of sexual fluids leads to diminished vital energy. Though ejaculation usually refers to a man's discharge of semen during sexual intercourse, it can also refer to a woman's discharge of bodily fluids during lovemaking.

The following exercise is a companion to the Five Tibetans, the purpose of which is to prevent depletion of vital energy due to loss of sexual fluids. The Tibetans recommended this exercise to be used by celibates to control sexual urges, prevent ejaculation, and move sexual energy up the spine, transmuting it into spiritual power. I want to make it abundantly clear that I do not personally recommend such a course. If you are celibate and that lifestyle suits you, then this exercise will relieve tension and enable you to deal more effectively with accumulated energy. For the majority of us who are sexually active, I include this exercise because it is valuable in strengthening the sex glands, thereby enhancing sexual activity. Some men may find this exercise helps in controlling ejaculation, thus enabling them to last longer during intercourse. In short, this exercise offers benefits to all who practice, whether they are celibate or not.

THE "SIXTH TIBETAN"

⊕

Stand up straight with your hands on your hips and your feet about four inches apart (figure 11). In this position, take a long, full, deep breath, inhaling through the nose. Then exhale through the mouth with your lips pursed in an "O." Bend forward as you exhale, leaning on your knees with your hands (figure 12).

In this forward position squeeze every bit of breath out of the trunk, until the abdomen is tightly pulled in. While holding the breath out and the abdomen in, return to a fully upright position with your hands on your hips (figure 13). Keep holding the breath out for several seconds. Then take in a long, slow, deep breath and relax.

Repeat this exercise a maximum of three times. Finish standing with your feet together and hands on your hips (figure 2). Take two full, deep breaths, inhaling through the nose and exhaling through the mouth, with your lips pursed in an "O."

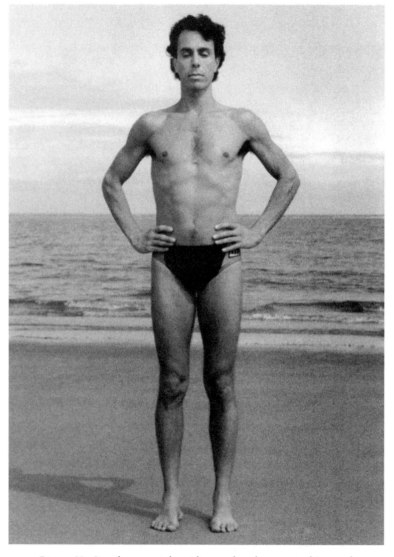

Figure 11. Stand up straight with your hands on your hips and
your feet about four inches apart. In this position,
take a long, full, deep breath, inhaling through the nose.
Then exhale through the mouth with your lips pursed in an "O."

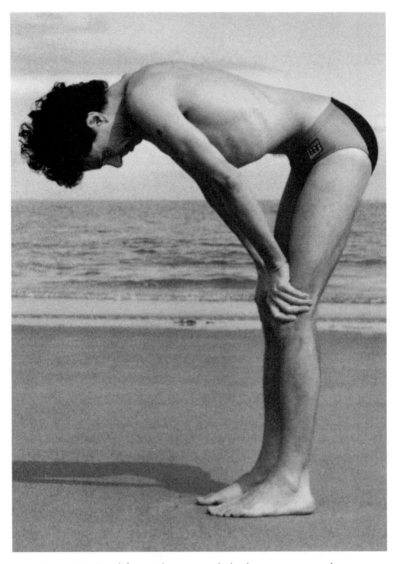

Figure 12. Bend forward as you exhale, leaning on your knees
with your hands. In this forward position squeeze every bit
of breath out of the trunk, until the abdomen is tightly pulled in.

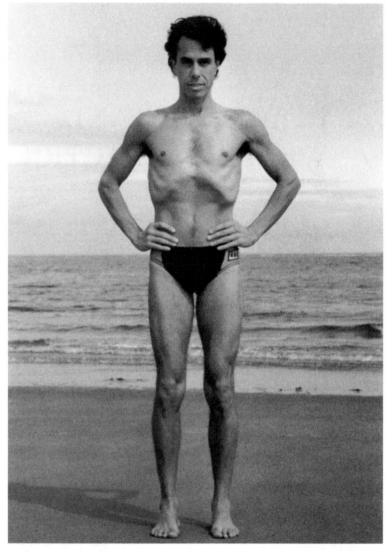

Figure 13. While holding the breath out and the abdomen in, return to a fully upright position with your hands on your hips. Keep holding the breath out for several seconds. Then take in a long, slow, deep breath and relax.

7 HOW, WHEN, AND WHERE TO PRACTICE

The short version of this chapter would simply read: "Practice the Five Tibetans anytime, anywhere. You will benefit from doing so." That is true. Nonetheless, there are conditions that will make your practice easier, more comfortable, and energetically optimal.

TIME OF DAY

You can practice the Five Tibetans anytime at all, but for best results I recommend practicing them in the morning before breakfast or in the evening before retiring to bed. I prefer to practice first thing in the morning, after showering, because these exercises give a good energetic edge to the day, which I find immensely valuable. Practicing the Five Tibetans at night usually brings on a deeper sleep and may cut down on the amount of time that you need to sleep. However, some people find that they get so energized after practicing these exercises that they can't get to sleep, and wind up in bed staring at the ceiling. You'll have to experiment to determine your preference. If you are really enthusiastic about the Five Tibetans, you can practice them in the morning *and* evening.

IS CLEANLINESS
REALLY NEXT TO GODLINESS?

Whether cleanliness is a primary criterion for divinity is questionable; however, being clean for your practice of the Five Tibetans is a good idea. I prefer to shower before practice, although some people sweat so much that they choose to shower afterward. At the very least, wash your face and hands in preparation for your practice.

Your yoga practice will feel more special if you prepare yourself by cleaning your body beforehand. It's a way of bringing an extra bit of attention to practice, in the same way as one dresses up for church. There's really no law prohibiting a person from wearing shorts and an old T-shirt to church, but there is something about putting on your best, cleanest clothes that adds an extra dimension of reverence. Since everything we do involves one mind-set or another, putting yourself in a state of mind in which your practice feels special is beneficial to your experience.

PRACTICE ON AN EMPTY STOMACH

It is best to practice the Five Tibetans no sooner than three hours after eating. You can get nauseated if you practice them on a full stomach. When you have a belly full of food, a lot of blood and circulatory energy is concentrated in the digestive organs. You want to liberate your circulation for yoga practice, letting blood flow freely throughout the entire body.

TEMPERATURE AND AIR

Whenever possible, practice in a place that is neither too hot nor too cold and is well ventilated.

DRESS FOR SUCCESS

Wear loose, nonrestrictive clothing, preferably made of cotton. The less clothing the better. Practicing in minimal clothing gives you greater freedom of movement.

WHERE TO PRACTICE

If possible, set aside a space solely for yoga practice. If this is not feasible, make sure to keep the place where you practice neat and clean. It is best to practice on a mat or a rug rather than on a hard surface.

AN ATTITUDE OF GRATITUDE

As much as you can, let your yoga practice be a special time, a time when you bring extra care and attention to what you do. Because they deliver so many benefits to overall health and well-being, the Five Tibetans are to be treasured and regarded with care and respect. You will enhance your overall experience by engaging in practice with a positive, grateful attitude.

⊕

Unlike many other forms of exercise or personal pursuit, practice of the Five Tibetans requires no special equipment, no particular setting, no particular type of weather, and nobody but yourself. By observing the few simple guidelines given here, you will find it easy to practice and experience the benefits offered by these unique exercises.

8 YOGANIDRA

One of the essential things to learn in the practice of yoga is the art of deep relaxation. For most people who embark upon stress-reduction programs, biofeedback courses, or relaxation classes, simply learning to relax is the goal. For a yogi, deep relaxation is both an essential ability in and of itself and a doorway to far greater endeavors, including conscious sleep, self-healing, and exploring the vast unknown. These abilities, rooted in the practice of deep relaxation, are all part of the process known as *yoganidra*. Known as the yogic sleep, yoganidra is attunement with and command over the energetic forces that course through the body and that are part of a universal energetic ocean.

DEEP RELAXATION

The primary key to yoganidra is learning to relax in a deep and profound manner. Having taught yoga classes for over two decades, I know just how hard something as simple as relaxing can actually be. I have watched yoga students fret and fidget and tense and hold themselves in a state of high anxiety when they were supposed to be relaxing. Relaxing, though it is a volitional process, involves giving up control, letting go, surrendering tension. You cannot relax and maintain tight control at the same time, but you *can* relax voluntarily, maintaining a state of alertness and lucidity of consciousness while your body seems to slip away. Deep relaxation involves a measure of trust. You have to be willing to let go of tension and believe that you will be all right.

To begin practicing deep relaxation, do the following: Put yourself in corpse pose, lying flat on your back with your legs fully extended and feet about twelve inches apart. Your arms are also outstretched, palms up, with hands about a foot away from your body (figure 14). Your eyes are closed. Make sure that you are warm enough and that your clothing is loose and nonrestrictive. In this position, practice long, slow breathing. With every exhalation let your body settle deeper into the ground, as though the force of gravity were increasing.

After a couple of minutes you can begin a systematic relaxation exercise. Start by bringing your attention to your feet. Breathing slowly and easily, feel your feet as fully as you can. As the breath flows in and out, consciously let go of any tension in your feet. Then move your attention to your lower legs. With every easy breath, let the muscles in your lower legs relax completely. Repeat this process with your knees, thighs, pelvis, lower abdomen, buttocks and lower back, mid-abdomen and mid-back, chest and upper back, upper arms, forearms, hands, neck, and face. At every part of your body, take as much time as you need to apply your attention fully to that area. If you are slow and careful and systematic, you will be amazed by how deeply relaxed you can get.

After you have systematically gone through your entire body, consciously relaxing every part, let your breath become as soft and gentle as possible. Let your attention rest on the breath in a feather-light manner. Do not apply intense concentration; just pay

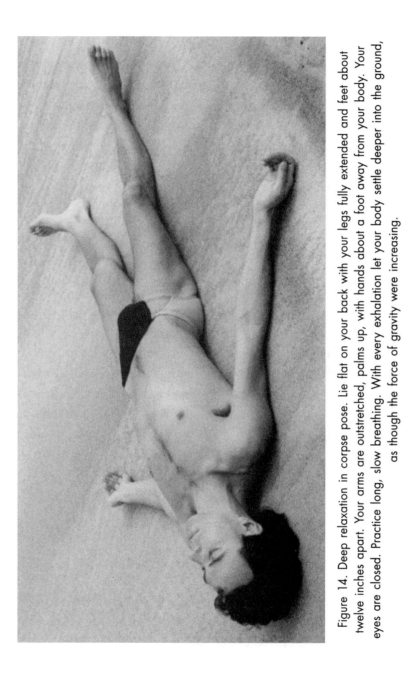

Figure 14. Deep relaxation in corpse pose. Lie flat on your back with your legs fully extended and feet about twelve inches apart. Your arms are outstretched, palms up, with hands about a foot away from your body. Your eyes are closed. Practice long, slow breathing. With every exhalation let your body settle deeper into the ground, as though the force of gravity were increasing.

attention in the easiest possible way. At first this may seem hard to do, but with practice you will get the hang of it.

At this point, you may drift off to sleep. There's no harm in that at all. Many people find that going through the progressed relaxation process just described is an excellent prelude to a good night's sleep. Especially if you are a very tense person, relaxing and then passing into sleep may be exactly what you need to do in your initial practice of yoganidra. Practice this deep relaxation technique daily for at least a month or two before going on to the next stages.

CONSCIOUS SLEEP

The next stage of yoganidra is a little more difficult than the first. It involves going through the entire progressed relaxation process as described, but keeping your mind fully awake and alert the whole time. This is difficult at first because most people associate lying down and relaxing with going to sleep. So there is an act of will involved here. You must pay close attention to the subtle ways that your body is releasing, but at the same time you must hang on to a wakeful core—a part of your mind that stays clear and aware—without falling asleep.

If you can put yourself into a profoundly deep relaxation and keep an alert mind, then sooner or later you will make the startling discovery that your body is actually completely asleep, but you are awake! I discovered this in a comical way. Because I occasionally snore lightly when I sleep on my back, the first time I slept with my mind awake I thought it was the funniest thing in the world to lie there and listen to my body's light, snoozing sounds.

Developing the ability to sleep consciously is a way to begin gaining voluntary control over involuntary functions. If you proceed deeply into the practice of yoga, you will find over time that you can voluntarily change your blood pressure, brain waves, heartbeat, and many other supposedly involuntary bodily processes. There are life-extending and energy-enhancing advantages to consciously controlling these functions. Developing the ability to sleep consciously is essential to the next stages of yoganidra. It may take you months to become adept at this practice, but if you apply yourself you will find that you can put your body to sleep, keep your mind in a relaxed meditative state, and wake yourself in ten or twenty minutes, feeling deeply rested and refreshed, as if you took a nap and meditated.

SELF-HEALING

Once you have found the way into a deep and profoundly relaxed state in which your mind is fully alert, you are ready to learn self-healing. There is an adage that states, "If you can feel it, you can move it." This is a fundamental principle of self-healing. Let's say that you are suffering from sinus congestion and a sore throat. After you have put yourself into a deeply relaxed state, as described earlier, place your awareness on your sinuses and throat, paying very close attention to how you feel there. Take time, perhaps several minutes, to thoroughly feel those areas. Without trying to force anything, simply intend that those areas will be restored to proper, healthy function. Keep your concentration easy; do not try to force anything. Just intend for healing to take place, simply and matter-of-factly. Then pay attention to your sensations, without forcing the issue further.

This is where control over the energetic currents of the body comes into play. If you are in a state of profound relaxation, then one very well-directed intention is enough to alter the energy flowing through your body and to reestablish a condition of health. This may sound simple, and it is. But do not confuse simple with easy. You must be in a profoundly relaxed state; if not, you will try this method and assume that it doesn't work. You must be so relaxed that there is no tension interfering with your mental intention for the restoration of health and balance. Health, after all, is a state of dynamic energy, balance, and vitality. It is a condition of dynamic well-being, not just the absence of disease. One of the things that any accomplished yogi understands is that the health of the body can be manipulated and directed by a well-focused mind. You will find through proper practice of the yoganidra method of healing that you will be able to positively alter your health in times of sickness or pain. You may not effect a total cure, but you will be able to make your condition appreciably better and more comfortable. Practice is the key. If you put in the time to train yourself well, you will be surprised by just how much self-healing you can accomplish. It is a wonderful, self-empowering act.

EXPLORING THE UNKNOWN

Beyond relaxation, beyond conscious sleep, and beyond self-healing lies the unknown. I can say precious little about it except this. We all live in the world with a sense of normalcy, a belief that things are a certain way and that there is some predictability to life. And this is largely true. Grass grows long and green instead of in purple squares, and the sun appears and disappears every day. So, in a sense, there is some predictability to life, but that predictability belies the immense mystery that is all around us.

After learning all the previous stages of yoganidra you are prepared for experiences I simply can't predict, because only you will go there, and the experiences will be yours, not mine. I can say that I have been to some pretty wild places, if they are "places" at all. I have been surrounded by blazing blue and orange fire, have encountered deities and beings of all kinds, and have shot through long, twined double-helix strands of DNA to realms that I can't

describe because I simply don't have words to fit those journeys.
I have witnessed what appear to be galaxies arising from the inky
black nothingness of deep space and dissolving again into nothingness, as though billions of years could be condensed into minutes
of experience.

The key to adventure travel in yoganidra is to develop the
ability to surrender. Truth be known, no matter how relaxed you
are, you may find yourself automatically tensing up if you begin
to shoot through a long, brightly lit tunnel at ultra-high speed.
That's perfectly understandable. You may decide at that moment
that such adventures are simply not for you. But if your sense of
curiosity and adventure outweighs your fears and sense of panic
in the face of overwhelming and often bizarre experiences, then
letting go is essential to going further. I help myself to get through
wild yoganidra explorations by remembering that the universe is
a friendly place. It is. Sure, there's plenty of danger too. But the
universe is fundamentally supportive, not hostile. Knowing this
helps.

Yogic scriptures are filled with intimations of these kinds of
experiences, but the accounts are not the experiences themselves.
The map is not the territory. What will happen to you, and where
you will go if you allow yourself, is something only you will find out.
If you practice yoganidra you will be as prepared as you can be for
some wild, wonderful adventures in inner space. We live in a great
big universe with parallel realities and countless other realms, beings,
and states than those we typically encounter during waking, sleeping, and dreaming. Since you live here, you might as well go out and
poke around a bit.

9 KUNDALINI MEDITATION

To use a somewhat shopworn but nonetheless accurate expression, meditation is not what you think. Meditation is beyond thought, beyond our typical experiences of waking, sleeping, and dreaming. At the same time though, one can be in meditation while in these daily states. Meditation is utterly straightforward, yet the process of meditation is also mysterious in what it reveals when we practice. It is immediately available; anyone can sit down and begin to meditate. Yet meditation is also something cultivated over a lifetime, like a pearl that accumulates from one irritating grain of sand. Meditation exists on the filamentous line between negative and positive, between the known and unknown. It begins as a practice, a technique, and over time becomes indistinguishable from all else. It is of this world, yet also opens us up to other worlds. Meditation is both a method and an all-pervasive way of being.

There are hundreds of meditation techniques originating from traditions that span the full spiritual spectrum. In all their various forms, meditation methods clarify the mind, expand awareness, and create inner harmony. There is no single ultimate technique of meditation; instead, different practices are temperamentally suited to particular individuals. At the same time, most methods will yield benefits for anyone who will invest time and energy in them. With meditation, practice is essential. Meditation is not like a piece of pie. You can't nibble off a little and decide whether it is good or not. It takes time and energy and concentration and regular practice to discover the power and value of any valid form of meditation. Casual flirtations with meditation will do little but create the effect of being at a spiritual smorgasbord. Only persistence yields the rewards of meditation practice.

Sensational occult literature has propagated wild expectations about meditation, promising that it will somehow lift you from the confines of your mortal form, rocket you from the face of the planet, and send you skittering off into vast other realms of experience to commune with angels and disembodied spooks. It's not that any of these things can't happen, but the truth is that *any expectations at all* are the bane of meditation practice, because expectations are mental abstractions. By contrast, the meditative mind is a brilliant mirror, finely polished and carrying no images of its own, that superbly reflects whatever appears before it. Through meditation, you become distinctly aware of every moment and stay present, right here, right now, moment by moment. Yes, meditation can stir up a lot of energy, and it does lead to extraordinary states of consciousness and experience. But fundamental to accessing states of superordinary awareness is to suspend expectation, to anticipate nothing, to dispense with preconceived notions. This is admittedly harder to do than to recommend.

Meditation works very differently from thinking. When thinking, the mind is filled with symbols—visual images, words, or other mental products that describe life in some way. But meditation involves dipping into the vast and limitless pool of pure consciousness, beyond abstraction and symbols. Meditation experiences such as visions and sensations of great energy come by clearing the mind, not by wishing and hoping for them. It is somewhat paradoxical. By suspending thought and abstraction, there is room for experiences to spontaneously occur, arising out of the eternal ebb and flux of energy and intelligence. These experiences, as interesting and alluring as they may be, are just more stuff, more phenomena. In and of themselves they are nothing special or significant. They are certainly not the end products of meditation. The real meditative benefit is a clear, burnished mind.

A friend of mine was once at a long and intensive meditation retreat. Over the course of a few weeks he had many unusual and powerful experiences. He felt as though he were floating in space, as though he were as big as a planet, as though he could embrace all of creation. There were times when he drifted out of his body and other times when sensations of energy roared up his spine. He was very excited about the experiences he was having, so he went to the teacher who was leading the retreat and recounted everything that had happened to him. After my friend was done giving a detailed rundown of all that had transpired, the teacher looked at him with a warm and reassuring smile and said, "Don't worry, it will pass." This is the full value of meditation experiences. They are like signs along a road. They are not the goal, just part of the scenery. They are interesting, but they are not what practice is about. It is only clear, pure mind that matters.

To derive the most from meditation, make time for daily practice, and do not hurry. No matter how much time you set aside to meditate, let that be a time when you are undisturbed by telephones, conversation, or other external distractions. You will encounter enough internal distractions to keep you well occupied, fighting for a little bit of clarity. Initially you will find that it is easier to meditate on an empty stomach. This is because after a full meal, blood circulation in the digestive organs is at an all-time high, making it hard to concentrate. While you can meditate at any time, it is often easiest to set aside time in the morning upon waking or in the evening prior to bed.

As with yoga practice, wear loose, nonrestrictive clothing, and meditate in a comfortable place. If you can, meditate in a natural setting such as the woods or the beach. Nature has a wonderful way of facilitating meditation because we come from nature, and it is a huge part of who and what we are. Wherever you meditate, keep that place neat, clean, and attractive. If you can, afford yourself a special spot for meditation only, even if it's just a small corner of a room. Create a mood by honoring that place. Keep flowers there. Recognize your meditation place as a special spot.

The following methods comprise a full practice of kundalini meditation. Each of the practices works to open the channels of the human energy system, liberating the flow of kundalini. Kundalini meditation practice burns away obstructions in energy flow, providing the mind with the monumental energy needed to be fully attentive to the present moment. Remember, the purpose of meditation is not to accumulate a bunch of fantastic experiences, even though they probably will come over time. Instead, the purpose is to bring enough attention to the present that the mind is brilliantly, vividly clear and dynamically awake and aware. Meditation enables us to live fully and completely in the moment, and that's all.

There are four meditation methods carefully described here; each practice builds upon the one before it. My recommendation is that you start by practicing the first method daily for at least a month or more before adding the second. Practice those in combination for at least that amount of time, then add the third. Again, practice for at least a month before adding the fourth technique. There is no value whatsoever in hurrying along and trying to engage in all the methods at once. Learning to practice correctly is essential, and that takes time.

CHAKRA MEDITATION

This is where we start with kundalini meditation. This method takes about half an hour to practice correctly, though you should feel free to meditate for longer if you are comfortable doing so.

Seat yourself comfortably in a cross-legged position. Full lotus is ideal, though it is typically too uncomfortable for most people. Any cross-legged position is fine, provided you keep your spine as erect as possible. You may wish to use a small pillow to raise yourself and make it easier to sit erect. Place hands on your knees. Eyes are closed, mouth is closed. The tip of your tongue should touch your upper palate.

In this position, breathe steadily and easily through the nose for several minutes. As you do this, release any tension in your muscles except for what you need to sit upright with a straight spine. Let your shoulders, abdomen, and facial muscles be very relaxed. Let your mind settle down as much as possible as you breathe. Throughout this meditation, breathing is a key element. It is not necessary to breathe long and deep, but the breath is steady and even, slightly deeper than a normal, relaxed breath. Maintain this breathing throughout the entire meditation.

Then direct your attention to the first chakra, muladhara, at the perineum, the spot at the very base of the spine between the anus and the genitals. Focus your attention there for about three minutes or so while breathing slowly and steadily. With every breath, feel as though you are breathing right through that center of energy. As much as possible, feel that place in your body. Let it be fully relaxed so you are not creating unnecessary tension.

From there, move your attention to the second chakra, svadhisthana, located at the lower spine at the level of the sex organs. Focus your attention at that spot for three minutes or so while breathing slowly and steadily. Again, with every breath, feel as though you are breathing right through that center of energy. As much as possible, feel that place in your body. The next point of attention is the third chakra, manipura, located along the spine at the area of the solar plexus. Focus your attention there for three minutes or so while breathing slowly and steadily. With every breath, feel as though you are breathing right through that center of energy, through the solar plexus and the spine. As much as possible, feel that place in your body.

Focus next on the fourth chakra, anahata, located at the spine directly opposite the center of the chest. Focus your attention there for three minutes or so while breathing slowly and steadily. With every breath, feel as though you are breathing right through the center of the chest and through that part of the spine. As much as possible, feel that place in your body.

Now bring your attention to the fifth chakra, visuddha, located at the spine across from the center of the throat. Focus your attention there for three minutes or so while breathing slowly and steadily. With every breath, feel as though you are breathing right through that center of energy. As much as possible, feel that place in your body.

Now bring your attention to the third eye, the sixth chakra—ajna—the spot at the root of the nose, between the eyebrows. Focus your attention there for three minutes or so while breathing slowly and steadily. With every breath, feel as though you are breathing right through the third eye, sending a beam of energy out in front of you. As much as possible, feel that place in your body.

From the third eye bring your attention to the crown chakra, sahasrara, at the top of the head. Focus your attention there for three minutes or so while breathing slowly and steadily. With every breath, feel as though you are breathing right through that center of energy. As much as possible, feel that place in your body, as though the entire top of your head is ablaze with energy.

From the crown chakra, bring your attention to the space all around your body, the aura. The aura is an energetic sheath that extends from the body in all directions. Focus your attention on that energetic sheath, extending outward from the body for at least a foot or more. With every breath, feel as though the aura is becoming increasingly concentrated with energy. As much as possible, feel that space all around you.

After you have brought your attention up through the chakras and to the aura, sit quietly, breathing slowly and steadily, allowing your entire system to assimilate the energy flow that results from this practice. Let your mind be as quiet and still as possible. Expect nothing, and do not try to provoke any particular experience. Instead, be as aware as you can of the moment, of your body posture, of the breath flowing in and out, of the feeling of the air around you, of the sights and smells of your surroundings. As vividly as you can, be aware of all that occurs without mentally latching on to any of it. It's all just phenomena; let it come and go with no effort of your own. Conclude your practice in this state of attention.

When you are done, take one or two long, deep breaths. Rub your hands together vigorously, then slowly rub them over your face as though you were washing yourself. Slowly open your eyes and relax for a minute or two before becoming more active.

This meditation opens up the chakra system, infusing it with energy. Steady breath and well-focused attention are critical to success. At each chakra, keep your attention as focused as possible. Avoid straying from the chakras. If you find your mind drifting away, bring your attention back to the center you are working on. Do not hurry. Take time to feel each center vividly.

Over time you will find it increasingly easy to feel those spots in the body, and to feel energy flowing through you.

SILVER CORD MEDITATION

After you have engaged in the chakra meditation for at least a month or more, you may wish to add this silver cord meditation. In the *Vigyana Bhairava Tantra*, one of the scriptural discourses of Siva, lord of the yogis, there is a description of this meditation. The silver cord is the central energy channel, sushumna, that runs up through the very center of the spine. The central channel is the energetic counterpart to the spinal cord, and as described in chapter 2 it is the course through which the kundalini energy flows.

Maintain the same position as before, sitting cross-legged with the spine erect, eyes shut, mouth closed, and the tip of the tongue touching the upper palate. Your hands are resting on your knees. The breath is steady and even. Start by meditating upon the chakras and the aura. After you have finished the chakra meditations, direct your full attention to your spine, feeling the entire length of it from the very base all the way up to the top of your neck. Take a few minutes to get fully into the feeling of your spine, much the same way as you would pay careful attention to the feeling of any other part of your body.

After a few minutes, picture a long silver cord running the entire length of the spine, directly through the center. The core of the silver cord is a vivid, crimson red. It is much like an insulated wire, with the silver cord the insulating material and the crimson red core a very fine wire inside. With every steady, even breath, concentrate your full attention on that silver cord with the bright red center. Picture it running from the base to the top of your spine. Feel your spine. Let your full attention reside there.

At first this meditation may seem a little simplistic. It is in fact extremely powerful and requires as much attention as you can possibly muster. As you hold the image of the silver cord with the crimson core firmly in your mind, the kundalini energy streams through the cord, energizing the entire chakra system. You start to expand—slowly at first, but then more rapidly. It is not uncommon to feel as though you contain within you the vastness of all space. Of course, as I said before, meditation experiences are not the goal. They are phenomena that flutter by. Nonetheless, a feeling of expansion is common and likely with this method, so you should know about it. You may also feel as though you are tapped into a limitless stream of energy.

Practice this method for as long as you like, and for just a little bit longer than is comfortable. It is always helpful to extend yourself beyond what is comfortable; there you play at the edge of your attention.

NAD YOGA MEDITATION

Now you have practiced the chakra meditation and the silver cord meditation. The next step is nad yoga. I recommend that you practice this in sequence after the first two methods we've already gone through so you'll have a lot of energy to work with. If you don't have that much time for meditation, this method can also be practiced by itself.

There are many phenomena that you will encounter as a result of meditation. One is the *nada,* or sound current. The nada is a vibrational current, a steady stream of sound that courses through absolutely everything. You are most likely to first encounter the sound current during meditation because it is at that time that the senses are most enlivened. You encounter the nada by hearing it. While the sound current is in fact hundreds or perhaps thousands of different sounds, you may initially hear it simply as one undifferentiated tone. The nada is best heard in a relatively quiet or sound-free environment. If you practice the chakra and silver cord meditations in a quiet place, you may hear a buzzing or humming in your head, especially near the right ear. This is not the sound of blood pumping; blood does not make a high-pitched whine as it flows. Nor should this sound be confused with Ménière's disease, a condition that causes vertigo and a loud ringing in the ears. What you hear is the sound current, a simple, seemingly innocuous tone that is an audible highway to the infinite.

At the end of the chakra and silver cord meditations you can either continue to sit erect, or else lie down. Either way, it is important to stay as alert as possible, because this method requires well-honed concentration. Falling asleep is therefore not desirable. If you lie down, do so on a flat surface without a pillow. Keep your legs straight and uncrossed, with your arms close to your sides and the palms of your hands turned upward. Your eyes and mouth are closed, and the tip of the tongue rests against the upper palate. Relax as much as you can, loosening muscular and mental tension. It is ideal to practice in a quiet, dark place. Late at night or early in the morning are excellent times for this practice, because the world is relatively still. If environmental noise is an unavoidable problem, use earplugs.

Turn all your attention to the inside of your head and listen closely. Concentrate initially on the right side of the head, near the inner ear. There will be some sort of sound there. You may hear a light ringing, a soft buzzing, or something akin to a faint rumble. Listen as closely as you can to whatever you hear, with absolute attention. Listen as carefully as you would if you were trying to hear someone who is in another room speaking at a whisper. Concentrate intently.

As you listen the sound will grow louder and will start becoming not one sound but many sounds together. In fact, you may hear so many sounds that the original one you heard may be lost. That's fine. As the sounds become louder, pick just one and focus on it. It doesn't matter which one you choose, but choose one and stay with it. Concentrate intently on that sound, much like concentrating on the sound of one instrument in a symphony. It will become steadily louder, and you may begin to feel that sound coursing through your entire body. As you listen with great concentration, the sound you are following may change into something else, something subtle and more refined. That's fine. Just go with it and keep your attention as focused as possible.

There are many sounds that you might hear, including ringing bells, flutelike tones, falling water, buzzing, the sound of the ocean, and sounds like crickets and birds. As you continue to practice this method you will hear ever more subtle sounds and rare tones. However, it is critical to pay very close attention, or the sounds will quickly fade away.

Here is how Siva, lord of the yogis, describes the sound current and meditation upon it in the *Siva Samhita:**

The first sound is like the hum of the honey-intoxicated bee. Next that of a flute, then of a harp; after this, by the gradual practice of yoga, the destroyer of the darkness of the world, he hears the sounds of ringing bells; then sounds like the roar of thunder. When one fixes full his attention on this sound, being free from fear, he gets absorption, O my beloved!

When the mind of the yogi is exceedingly engaged in this sound, he forgets all external things, and is absorbed in this sound.

---

*Rai Bahadur Srisa Chandra Vasu, *The Siva Samhita* (New Delhi: Oriental Books Reprint Corporation, 1979).

By this practice of yoga he conquers all the three qualities (i.e., good, bad and indifferent); and being free from all states, he is absorbed in chidakas (the ether of intelligence).

When you meditate on the sound current, you attune your attention first to the sound itself and eventually to the source of the sound. With practice you will find yourself merging with the sound current so fully that there is no way to differentiate where you end and the sound begins. You will go through many altered states and find yourself in a heightened state of awareness. Remember, what this is all about is liberating energy so you can bring acute and well-honed attention to the moment. Phenomena, however dazzling and rich, will come and go.

The experience of the nada is like nothing else. The only way to understand what it is like to listen to the sound current is to practice. Nothing else will do. The sounds you will hear are like no others. To find your entire being bathed in the rare vibrations of the sound current is as sweet and exquisite an experience as you can have. The key to success with this method, as with all methods, is persistence and the dogged pursuit of complete attention. You will find that the sounds are very slippery. They come and they go, they disappear, they change, they diminish, they roar.

Practice the sound current meditation for at least fifteen minutes. Longer is better, because it is valuable to push your own ability to concentrate and stay alert. After practicing, relax for a few minutes.

The mind is like a serpent, forgetting all its unsteadiness by hearing the nada, it does not run away anywhere.*

---

*Pancham Sinh, *The Hatha Yoga Pradipika* (New Delhi: Oriental Books Reprint Corporation, 1980).

NAD YOGA AND THE CENTRAL CHANNEL

The final step of this kundalini meditation is a fusion of methods. Following your practice of the chakra and silver cord meditations, remain in a sitting position and begin meditation on the sound current. After a few minutes of tapping into the sound current, put your attention simultaneously on the central channel running up through the spine. It is not necessary to visualize the silver cord, just feel that channel running up through the spine at the same time that you are listening to the sound current. Listen intently to the sound current and feel the central channel. You will find that you can do both.

Assuming that you have taken time to cultivate good meditation habits, and assuming that you are applying your attention as fully as possible, you will find this to be an extraordinary meditation. Concentration on the central channel plugs your attention into the core of your energy system, while concentration upon the sound current taps you into the source of all energy and intelligence. The fusion is very powerful. This method has the capacity to liberate a massive flow of energy, circulating it through your entire being. Practice for at least fifteen minutes following the chakra and silver cord meditations, and increase the time as you are able. You will find that over time you will easily feel tapped into the source of all energy. That is exactly where you want to be.

WHERE DO YOU GO FROM HERE?

It's a lovely thing to admire a mountain from afar, and quite another to scale it and stand at the summit, having exerted yourself and gone beyond your personal comfort zone. Similarly, it can be interesting to read about the Five Tibetans and various forms of meditation, and to think about the energetic flow of the body/mind and the vastness of human potential. But it is quite another thing to practice the methods described in this book. Reading about these yogic methods of power is a lot like sightseeing. Until you really get into them, until you make them part of your life, they're just more scenery in an ever-shifting landscape.

If you feel any affinity at all for the methods described here, then practice them. You don't need to find a guru, an ashram, or anything else to get started. Go through the instructions carefully, step by step, and make these methods part of your life. Reading about them is enjoyable; practicing them is enlivening and enlightening. The Five Tibetans are rare methods. They offer many benefits for relatively little time and exertion. These exercises, coupled with kundalini meditation, constitute a powerful yoga practice that can literally change your life, if you let it.

BEYOND METHOD

As I have said previously, the purpose of engaging in various kundalini meditation practices is not to accumulate a load of extraordinary experiences but to generate as much energy as possible, bringing your full attention to that endeavor so as to experience the present moment vividly and fully alive. If you faithfully practice the sequence of methods described here you will generate immense energy, liberating the kundalini force and circulating that energy through your entire body/mind. Through meditation practice, you will sharpen your attention to the point that you will indeed be able to keep focused on the moment, which is the only time there is. Right here, right now is the only time we can ever live. Nobody ever lives yesterday or tomorrow; we do all our living right here. By bringing immense energy and well-honed attention to the moment, we can be fully and brilliantly aware. This way of being is beyond method. It is not a technique, it is simply being. All the contortions of yoga—all the breathing, the concentration, the exercises, the diligent practice—bring us eventually to the point where there is nothing at all to be done, nothing to grasp at, nothing to pursue, no goal to attain, just the sheer immensity of being right here, right now, the only time there is.